Pathophysiology of Nursing

DeMYSTiFieD

Notice

Medicine is an ever-changing science. As new research and clinical experience broaden our knowledge, changes in treatment and drug therapy are required. The authors and the publisher of this work have checked with sources believed to be reliable in their efforts to provide information that is complete and generally in accord with the standards accepted at the time of publication. However, in view of the possibility of human error or changes in medical sciences, neither the authors nor the publisher nor any other party who has been involved in the preparation or publication of this work warrants that the information contained herein is in every respect accurate or complete, and they disclaim all responsibility for any errors or omissions or for the results obtained from use of the information contained in this work. Readers are encouraged to confirm the information contained herein with other sources. For example and in particular, readers are advised to check the product information sheet included in the package of each drug they plan to administer to be certain that the information contained in this work is accurate and that changes have not been made in the recommended dose or in the contraindications for administration. This recommendation is of particular importance in connection with new or infrequently used drugs.

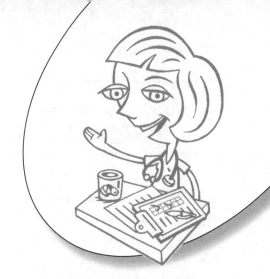

Pathophysiology of Nursing

DeMYSTiFieD

Helen Christina Ballestas, PhD, RN, ANP-BC
Assistant Professor of Nursing
Adelphi University
Garden City, New York

Carol Caico, PhD, CS, WHNP-BC
Assistant Professor of Nursing
New York Institute of Technology, Old Westbury
Seaford, New York

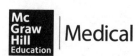 Medical

New York   Chicago   San Francisco   Athens   London   Madrid
Mexico City   Milan   New Delhi   San Juan   Singapore   Sydney   Toronto

Pathophysiology of Nursing/Demystified

Copyright © 2014 by The McGraw-Hill Companies, Inc. All rights reserved. Printed in the United States of America. Except as permitted under the United States Copyright Act of 1976, no part of this publication may be reproduced or distributed in any form or by any means, or stored in a data base or retrieval system, without the prior written permission of the publisher.

2 3 4 5 6 7 8 9 0 DOC/DOC 18 17 16

ISBN 978-0-07-177202-0
MHID 0-07-177202-2

This book was set in Berling by Thomson Digital.
The editor was Brian Kearns.
The production supervisor was Richard Ruzycka.
Project Management was provided by Shaminder Pal Singh, Thomson Digital.
The cover illustration is by Lance Lekander.
RR Donnelley was printer and binder.

This book is printed on acid-free paper.

Library of Congress Cataloging-in-Publication Data

Ballestas, Helen Christina, author.
  Pathophysiology of nursing demystified / Helen Christina Ballestas, Carol Caico.
    p. ; cm.
  Includes bibliographical references and index.
  ISBN 978-0-07-177202-0 (pbk. : alk. paper) — ISBN 0-07-177202-2 (pbk. : alk. paper)
  I. Caico, Carol, author. II. Title.
  [DNLM: 1. Disease—Handbooks. 2. Nursing Care—Handbooks. WY 49]
  RT49
  610.73—dc23
                                                    2013021107

McGraw-Hill books are available at special quantity discounts to use as premiums and sales promotions, or for use in corporate training programs. To contact a representative please e-mail us at bulksales@mcgraw-hill.com.

This book is dedicated to the two loves of my life, my grandsons Antonio and Nicholas.
You have given me the drive and dedication to see this project through.
Know that you are my constant inspiration in all that I do.
And also know that your "GAMA"
loves you both very much.

To my husband: you have travelled with me for such a long time
and still support me in everything I do, thank you and I love you.

To my children: Monica, you are my oldest and closest friend.
Daniel, my one and only son, you truly are the light of
my life, and Elisa, you keep me young and smiling.

To my nursing students: What can I say, without all of you, I would be nothing.
Thank you for teaching me so many lessons. I am the teacher, nurse,
and nurse practitioner today because you have
supported me in so many ways.

—Helen Christina Ballestas

I thank my husband Nick who supports all my endeavors with love.
I thank my four wonderful grandchildren, Hayden, Avery, Harrison and
Ella who keep me happy and grounded. My sons and
wonderful daughter-in-laws graciously give me support.
I continue to enjoy teaching and preparing students to
become the best RN's possible.

—Carol Caico

Contents

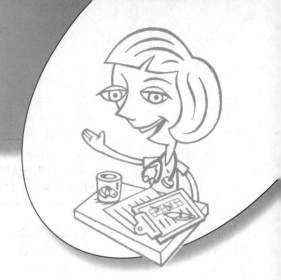

Introduction

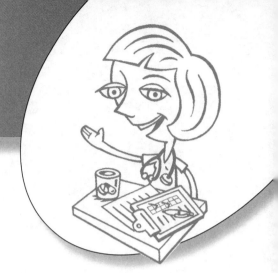

Nurses lead very busy and complicated lives. The work we do is exhausting yet rewarding. Nursing and medicine change continuously, and as professionals, it is our responsibility to move with the flow of change.

This book was envisioned to be a synopsis of major topics currently seen in medicine. Its main objective was to have information at a glance so that nursing professionals can deliver safe patient care.

The target audience comprises nursing students, current working nurses, and nurse practitioners. In the nursing profession, the continuum of professional education has no ending.

Enjoy the book, read it when quick references are needed, and take care of your patients safely.

chapter 1

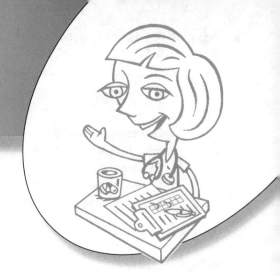

Neurologic System

Introduction

The neurological system is an intricate framework of cranial nerves, sensory and motor nerves, and peripheral and autonomic pathways that transfer information to and from the brain via the spinal column. The nerves necessary for overall human function lie close to one another in an intricate pattern for proper functioning.

Within the central nervous system lie the following: the meninges, the cerebral spinal fluid (CSF), the cerebral vasculature, and the brain (cerebrum, cortex, basal ganglia, diencephalon, thalamus, hypothalamus, brainstem, midbrain, pons, and medulla oblongata). Additionally, four integrated functional units responsible for gait and balance (equilibrium) lie here: the bulboreticular formation (balance), reticular activating system (responsible for sensory pathways), the limbic system (control emotions), and the sleep center.

Within the peripheral nervous system are the 12 pairs of cranial nerves (CN I–CN XII) and the 31 pairs of spinal nerves. The reflexes and the reflex pathways are integral part of the neurological system. Two major reflexes exist: the brain reflexes and the spinal cord reflexes. Pain sensation is modulated via the pain pathways that extend from the sensory cortex, through the thalamus, the midbrain, the medulla, and the spinal cord.

The system is fine-tuned, and when working well, it is responsible for almost every homeostatic response within the body. When there are problems within the nerves, the overall function of their neurotransmitters, the brain, the spinal column, or the pathways is profoundly disturbed. A delicate balance must always exist. Any type of brain assault or traumatic spinal cord injury affects the functioning of the body.

Cerebral Vascular Accidents (Stroke)

The brain is an extraordinarily powerful organ. In order to control and regulate all required systemic functions, the brain requires adequate perfusion. Important nutrients are delivered via the bloodstream to help synthesize all its important roles. There are times, however, when the blood flow is interrupted. Interruption can either be from an ischemic event (an event that is considered ischemic is one that occurs when there is insufficient blood flow to a particular area and that area begins to suffer the consequences, hence ischemia) or from occlusion due to a thrombus, plaque, or blood clot (embolic). Ischemic strokes include lacunar infarct, carotid circulation obstruction, or vertebrobasilar occlusion.

In addition, a stroke can occur when there is a hemorrhagic event within the tight walls of the cranial vault. Even small accumulations of blood create a potential problem that if unmanaged can also contribute to ischemia of the delicate brain tissues.

Hemorrhagic strokes include intracerebral hemorrhage, subarachnoid hemorrhage (SAH), intracranial hemorrhage, or arteriovenous malformations (AVMs).

Depending on the extent of damage in terms of time elapsed and tissue and location, strokes can have devastating results.

Ischemic strokes considered to be thrombotic in nature often warn with prior transient ischemic attacks (TIAs) that can last from minutes to hours, with quick resolution. Usually there is a temporary blockage that corrects itself. The patient feels some paresthesia, weakness, and slurred speech, which resolves spontaneously. It can occur during sleep time or upon awakening, most often in the morning hours. Common sites of occurrence include the carotid artery, the vertebral and basilar arteries, at the bifurcation of the middle cerebral artery, the anterior cerebral artery, or the posterior cerebral artery. Embolic strokes can also present with a TIA or without warning. The most common site is the middle cerebral artery. Usually these patients have a previous history of some sort of cardiovascular compromise such as myocardial infarction, congestive heart failure, problems with the heart valves and atrial fibrillation, bacterial endocarditis, or rheumatic endocarditis. Moreover, onset is sudden and devastating. Although the majority of embolic strokes are blood clots or plaque breakoffs, rarely the embolic event can also be induced from fat emboli, air emboli, or tumor cell emboli.

In ischemic stroke, cellular damage—often times irreparable—occurs within 10 seconds of cessation of crucial blood flow. Within a few minutes thereafter, neuron damage is pervasive. Surrounding the ischemic area, much like the epicenter of an earthquake, some viable tissue may remain. In addition, shifts in electrolytes, changes in ionic gradients, and inability of the mitochondria to produce adenosine triphosphate (ATP) needed for energy quickly manifests. Free radicals become rampant, affecting the all-important ion calcium from shifting back and forth from the cerebral cell. Because the body views the ischemic event as an inflammatory agent, edema aggregates and persists for 3 days after the event. Further, liquefaction occurs in the damaged tissue and this is due to hydrolytic enzymes released with cellular damage and debris.

Hemorrhagic strokes are bleeding episodes that occur deep within the brain parenchyma. Oftentimes, the patient has uncontrolled hypertension or an undiagnosed aneurysm that ruptures. Other times, there is an AVM deep within the circle of Willis in the brain. Berry aneurysms contribute to these strokes. These are small miniscule out-pouchings that rupture and cause devastation. These strokes are classified as intracerebral hemorrhage, subarachnoid hemorrhage, or aneurysms. Commonly, once there is a brain bleed, vasospasms occur along with edema because of the accumulating blood. If the accumulation of blood and its accompanying inflammatory response are severe enough, brain shifts or brain herniation can occur. Blood can seep into the ventricular system, where it is picked up with a lumbar tap. If the cerebral spinal fluid contains blood, it is one of the confirmatory diagnoses for hemorrhagic bleeds most specifically, subarachnoid hemorrhage (Figures 1–1 and 1–2).

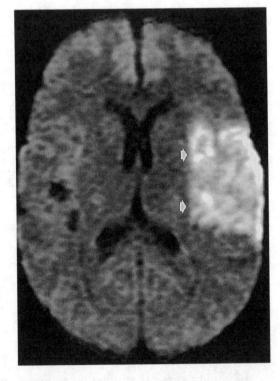

FIGURE 1–1 • Acute left MCA infarct on MRI of a 65 year-old hypertensive man. The MRI demonstrates increased signal intensity (arrows). Abnormalities in MRI occur before those seen on CT during ischemic strokes. (Reproduced with permission from Chen MYM, Pope TL Jr, Ott DJ, eds. *Basic Radiology.* New York, NY: McGraw-Hill; 2004:338.)

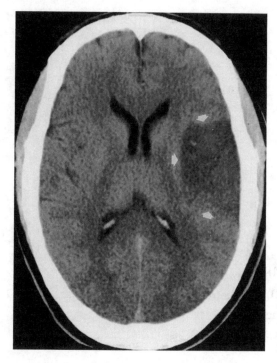

FIGURE 1–2 • Noncontrast CT image of a subacute left middle cerebral artery infarct (arrows). This was done 2 weeks after the stroke in the same patient as previous figure. CT findings occur later than MRI findings in ischemic strokes (Reproduced with permission from Chen MYM, Pope TL Jr, Ott DJ, eds. *Basic Radiology*. New York, NY: McGraw-Hill; 2004:338.)

Clinical Manifestations

- Amaurosis fugax = sudden but brief loss of eye vision
- Changes in vision that include bitemporal or hemianopia
- Changes in speech pattern
- Severe crushing headache
- Changes/disturbance in gait
- Paralysis: face, body, contralateral side of event
- Weakness especially to one side of the body
- Dizziness
- Confusion
- Nausea, projectile vomiting
- Vertigo
- Ataxia
- Coma
- Nuchal rigidity (SAH)
- Changes in level of consciousness

- Seizures (AVM)
- Pronator drift
- Positive Romberg sign
- Neurogenic bladder
- Dysarthria
- Apraxia

Diagnostic Tests

- Computed tomographic (CT) scan of the head
- Magnetic resonance imaging (MRI)
- Carotid studies
- Magnetic resonance angiography (MRA)
- Labs: complete blood count (CBC), sedimentation rate, blood glucose, cholesterol/lipid panel, homocysteine
- Lumbar puncture: cerebral spinal fluid (CSF) analysis
- Electrocardiogram (ECG)
- Electroencephalogram (EEG)
- Blood cultures

Treatment

If the event occurred because of a hypertensive episode with prolonged hypertension, treatment is focused on maintaining an acceptable blood pressure consistently. If the event occurred because of an aberrant cardiac rhythm such as atrial fibrillation, warfarin is started promptly. In addition, vigilance of cholesterol levels, good glycemic control, and smoking cessation are part of the treatment plan, as a patient with a stroke history has a higher incidence of re-stroking. If the event occurred because of occlusion with the carotid arteries, then re-vascularization is indicated. The overall approach is an interdisciplinary one where the physician, nurses, physical and occupational therapists, as well as respiratory and rehabilitation therapists are central to recovery if not, optimization of lifestyle to the best ability of the patient.

Nursing Interventions and Complications

In caring for patients with stroke, the nurse must keep in mind the multiple modifiable (prior history of stroke, smoking, atrial fibrillation [embolic possibility], diabetes, congestive heart failure, coronary artery disease [atherosclerosis], high cholesterol patterns, excessive alcohol and drug [cocaine] use, and nonmodifiable (advancing age, ethnicity, and gender) risk factors of stroke.

Safety and mobility are also paramount to monitor. Patients with reduced stamina, changes in range of motion, unilateral weakness, and alterations of their senses place them at risk for falls. Medication administration and patient teaching regarding the importance of adherence and compliance is critical for the nurse to focus on. Patients need to be reminded that medications for blood pressure and for atrial fibrillation are lifelong and although a stabilization of the blood pressure or heart rhythm will most likely occur, it means the medications are working and they must stay on them. Explaining to patients the importance of follow-up care should be reinforced.

Attention to supportive care is required of the nurse: physical therapy, occupational therapy, recreational therapy, rehabilitation nursing, social work involvement, psychology, and speech therapy (Table 1–1).

CLINICAL ALERT

Safety in terms of blood pressure management and control is a clinical alert that all nurses should focus on because the sequelae of poor blood pressure control carries a poor prognosis in a large brain bleed.

Dementia/Alzheimer

Dementia is an overall label for cognitive changes that occur almost exclusively among the gerontologic patient. Organic brain changes cause cognitive and intellectual impairment, inappropriate judgment, loss of ability to think abstractly, loss of reasoning skills, changes in memory (both remote and recent), and emotional instability. Many dementia patients can either be lethargic or aggressive. Progressive organic brain changes place the patient at risk for a host of complications, with safety, in general, being the most common problem. It is postulated that as the aging live longer, dementia cases will be common because patients older than age 75 years are mostly affected.

There are several types of dementia. One, for example, is dementia that can form after years of plaque buildup within the brain (atherosclerosis). Diffuse Lewy body dementia occurs when clumps of α-synuclein and ubiquitin protein

TABLE 1–1 Well-Documented Risk Factors for Stroke[a]

Nonmodifiable risk factors

Increased age
Male sex
Low birth weight
African American ethnicity
Family history of stroke

Modifiable risk factors

Vascular
  Hypertension (BP >140 mm Hg systolic or 90 mm Hg diastolic)
  Cigarette smoking
  Asymptomatic carotid stenosis (>60% diameter)
  Peripheral artery disease

Cardiac
  Atrial fibrillation (with or without valvular disease)
  Congestive heart failure
  Coronary heart disease

Endocrine
  Diabetes mellitus
  Postmenopausal hormone therapy (estrogen ± progesterone)
  Oral contraceptive use

Metabolic
  Dyslipidemia
    High total cholesterol (top 20%)
    Low HDL cholesterol (<40 mg/dL)
  Obesity (especially abdominal)

Hematologic
  Sickle cell disease

Lifestyle
  Physical inactivity

BP, blood pressure; HDL, high-density lipoprotein.
[a]Less well-documented modifiable risk factors include migraine with aura, metabolic syndrome, high alcohol consumption (≥5 drinks per day), drug abuse, sleep-disordered breathing, hyperhomocysteinemia, various hypercoagulability markers (e.g., anticardiolipin or antiphospholipid antibody), various inflammatory conditions or markers (e.g., periodontal disease or C-reactive protein), and various systemic infections (e.g., *Chlamydia pneumoniae* or cytomegalovirus).
Data from Goldstein LB, et al. Guidelines for the primary prevention of stroke. A guideline for healthcare professionals from the American Heart Association/American Stroke Association. *Stroke.* 2011;42:517-584.

in neurons aggregate. The most common dementia with this disorder is seen in patients with Parkinson disease and is only confirmed on autopsy.

Alzheimer dementia, a very common form of dementia, occurs insidiously and is progressive. There is significant loss of brain matter through degenerative processes. There is a small familial tendency, can occur in patients with previous head trauma, and with genetic testing, indicates presence of the apoE4 gene. In addition, patients who may have been exposed to viruses, lack acetylcholine in the brain, ingested excessive amounts of aluminum, developed accumulations of amyloid bodies, or developed neurofibrillary fibers can fall victim to the disorder. Although the etiology may exist genetically, it is not all conclusive and there are no specific tests to diagnose the disease.

Structural changes to the brain matter in Alzheimer disease occur most prominently within the hypothalamus, causing fissures to develop and the ventricles to enlarge. Additional areas of organic brain changes include the entorhinal cortex, association cortex, and the basal forebrain.

In general, there are three main courses of the disease, and it progresses over a period of years. The average life span after the initial diagnosis is made is approximately 8 years. Stage I considered the early stage lasts approximately 2–4 years. This is usually the time where the patient's family begins to notice changes. Stage II is considered the middle stage lasting 2–10 years. Sundowning; pronounced memory changes; restlessness; insomnia; difficulty writing, reading, and speaking; being suspicious; and hiding things are increasingly more noticeable. Stage III is the final stage lasting 1–2 years. The patient is unable to communicate with words and is unable to recognize loved ones. The patient forgets how to eat, bathe, use the toilet, ambulate, and swallow and oftentimes becomes bed-bound. They have no sense of time, fall often, and are susceptible to infections such as pneumonia. Falls, fractures, and seizures are common.

Continued care is required for these patients in a safe environment. Assistance with activities of daily living (ADLs), medication administration, healthcare providers appointments, vision/hearing care, and mobility are the main focus as the stages progress (Table 1–2).

Clinical Manifestations

- Memory loss/deterioration (STM)
- Lost in familiar surroundings
- Personality changes: combative, suspicious, inappropriate behaviors

TABLE 1–2 The Mini-Mental State Exam

Patient_____ Examiner_____ Date_____

Maximum	Score	
		Orientation
5	( )	What is the (year) (season) (date) (day) (month)?
5	( )	Where are we (state) (country) (town) (hospital) (floor)?
		Registration
3	( )	Name 3 objects: 1 second to say each. Then ask the patient all 3 after you have said them. Give 1 point for each correct answer. Then repeat them until he/she learns all 3. Count trials and record. Trials _____
		Attention and Calculation
5	( )	Serial 7's. 1 point for each correct answer. Stop after 5 answers. Alternatively spell "world" backward.
		Recall
3	( )	Ask for the 3 objects repeated above. Give 1 point for each correct answer.
		Language
2	( )	Name a pencil and watch.
1	( )	Repeat the following "No ifs, ands, or buts"
3	( )	Follow a 3-stage command: "Take a paper in you hand, fold it in half, and put it on the floor."
1	( )	Read and obey the following: CLOSE YOUR EYES
1	( )	Write a sentence.
1	( )	Copy the design shown.
	_____	Total score ASSESS level of consciousness along a continuum _____ Alert Drowsy Stupor Coma

Source: Neurologynerdsite (www.neurologynerdsite.com).

- Ataxia
- Cognitive impairment
- Apraxia
- Agnosia
- Poor judgment
- Loss of abstract thinking
- Acute confusion
- Weight loss
- Loss of ability to care for self
- Carelessness about personal appearances
- Speech impediments
- Incontinence

Diagnostic Tests

As mentioned earlier, there are no specific tests to rule in or out Alzheimer disease. Diagnosis is usually made on the basis of the symptomatology, progressive memory loss, and changes in the patient's overall psychosocial status. Upon death, the disease can be confirmed through an autopsy where areas of the brain are obtained looking for the neurofibrillary fibers and neuropathic sclerotic changes as well as the aggregation of proteins within the brain tissue.

Mental status is determined by application of the Mini Mental Examination, clinical assessment, age of onset, and absence of exposure to viruses or lack of head injury. CT scan and or an MRI are ordered to rule out brain pathology.

Treatment

There is no cure for Alzheimer dementia. However, there are medications available that help to slow the progression of the disease to some extent. Of the myriad of medications available to help slow down progression—cholinesterase inhibitors, memantine, and beta drugs that offer some level of neuroprotection—none can stop the disease process. Patients may be started on antidepressive medications or mood stabilizers. Care is focused on assisting with socializing skills as long as possible, promotion of sleep and rest, and respite care for the caregiver and family members who bear the brunt of this devastating disease's effects.

Nursing Interventions and Complications

Assist the patient in maintaining an optimal level of cognitive function. Activities such as reading, writing, sewing, and playing musical instruments are important. Reduce environmental stimuli because the patient is unable to process multiple actions and can be further confused. Be calm and approach your patient in a calm manner. Do not argue with or challenge the patient in any way because the patient may become overly aggressive. Introduce yourself to the nurse every time as the patient will not remember the nurse. Keeping the environment as safe as possible—removal of sharp objects, turning off the gas in gas stoves, double-bolting the doors with keys that are stored safely, and storing medications in a safe place—is vital. Patients with Alzheimer often do better in their own environment. Small pets and throw rugs and other household items should be cleared for safety and to avoid costly falls. Schedule consistency is best for this patient. Encourage patients to express their feelings and/or thoughts notwithstanding the inability to sometimes understand their speech because of speech problems that often accompany the disease process. As the disease progresses, assistive devices and specialty beds may be required in the home along with 24-hour-7-day-a-week care.

The nurse should offer respite care for the caregivers as well. Caregivers are sandwiched between the responsibilities of their jobs, toward their kids, and now aging ill parents.

Family members need to understand the pathologic progression of the disease process, remembering that at the last stage of dementia, patients may require extensive supportive care. Difficult decisions at end of life include whether to withhold nutrition and hydration, and the nurse is expected to support the family during this difficult time. If the decision is made to maintain nutrition and hydration, a feeding tube will be placed. Allow the patient's family to be equally involved in the care and decision-making process for the patient. This gives the family members a sense of control and involvement in the final wishes of the patient.

CLINICAL ALERT

Safety of the patient is paramount. In early disease, periods of lucidity interspersed with confusion are common. Family members may not always recognize the symptoms until well into stage II or after a fall, fracture, or other injury. Whether the patient is institutionalized or is cared for at home, focus should be on independence as long as possible and avoidance of injury in general.

Head Injury

Head injuries are categorized as traumatic and nontraumatic. Examples of traumatic injuries include motor vehicle/motorcycle accidents, skull fractures from blunt force trauma, concussion, contusions, and subdural hematomas. Other samples of traumatic brain injuries include factors that existed before that have now caused marked cerebral edema (vasogenic, cytotoxic, ischemic interstitial), cerebral hypoxia, or increased intracranial pressure (IICP) (with various etiologies). Nontraumatic brain injuries are categorized as injuries that occur secondary to stroke, transient ischemic attacks, hemorrhage, aneurysm rupture, herniation syndromes, or deformities of the AVM in the brain causing rupture and brain bleeding.

Within the cranial vault lie the delicate tissues of the brain. The skull consists of hard bony plates and fissures that surround the brain in a protective cocoon. Skin, hair, meninges, and cerebral spinal fluid provide additional protection. The protective tissues absorb the brunt of external forces; however, when the external forces are too great, there is brain damage or head injury. When there is a head injury, the cervical neck is protected until fractures or cervical separations are ruled out. Within this section of the neck lies the highest order of function within the human body.

Closed head injuries are defined as injuries that occur without a break in the skull's integrity. An acceleration–deceleration injury causes the brain to jolt forward and backward within the cranium. Nerve endings and tender tissues can be sheared resulting from the force of the trauma. The forward motion of the injury within the skull is called coup. As the head falls backward from deceleration forces, countercoup mechanics follow.

Open head injuries involve some degree of impaired skin integrity. The scalp, the meninges, and/or the brain tissues are involved. Open head injuries carry a high risk of infection. Types of skull fractures that expose the brain include linear fractures, depressed skull fractures, comminuted fractures, or basilar skull fractures.

After injury, neuroprotective enzymes, most specifically cytokines, are released. Various research studies have demonstrated that these brain-specific cytokines can offer information on brain injuries. Measurement of cytokines utilizing microdialysis has demonstrated promise at times of injury and gross overall cerebral inflammatory response (Figure 1–3).

Clinical manifestations are based on the type of injury. They are detailed below.

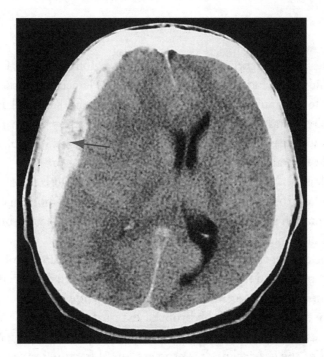

FIGURE 1–3 • CT scan of an acute subdural hematoma (arrow) seen as a hyperdense clot with an irregular border. There is a midline shift from the mass effect of the accumulated blood. (Reproduced with permission from Kasper DL, Braunwald E, Fauci AS, Hauser SL, Longo DL, Jameson JL. *Harrison's Principles of Internal Medicine.* 16th ed. New York: McGraw-Hill; 2005:2450.)

Skull Fractures

- Bone displacement
- Associated facial trauma
- Anosmia (loss of function cranial nerve [CN] I)
- Periorbital ecchymosis (raccoon eyes)
- Rhinorrhea (leakage of cerebral spinal fluid from the nose)
- Otorrhea (leakage of cerebral spinal fluid from the ears)
- Accumulating blood within the ear canal
- CN VII damage causing facial paralysis
- Progressive cardiopulmonary compromise

Coup Countercoup Injuries

- Coma
- Poor flexor and/or extensor responses

- Abnormal posturing
- Hemorrhage
- Progressive cardiopulmonary compromise

Concussion/Contusion

- Syncope
- Loss of consciousness (often thought of as a neuroprotective event in response to changes in pressure, sudden changes to the neurons of the brain, and ischemia)
- Amnesia post injury
- Dizziness
- Eventual sequelae that includes anxiety, impaired memory, and/or judgment as well as changes in memory
- Vital sign changes
- Pupillary response changes
- Motor response changes

Stroke

Clinical manifestations are detailed in the Ischemic and Hemorrhage Stroke sections.

Cerebral Edema, IICP

- Headache
- Changes in level of consciousness
- Nausea, vomiting
- Visual changes
- Papilledema
- Pupillary dilation
- Progressive cardiopulmonary compromise

Diagnostic Tests

- MRIs
- CT scan

- Lumbar puncture
- Blood work: there are no specific labs in head injuries, but blood work dictates inflammatory responses expected with severe injuries to the head

Treatment

Treatment is focused on mechanism of injury and sequelae of events. Medications to reduce cerebral edema such as mannitol or in some cases furosemide are indicated. When edema is severe, a shunt is placed deep within the skull to help reduce pressures that if allowed to continue may cause herniation syndrome.

Additional medications may include carbamazepine, phenytoin (for seizure management), diazepam (for prolonged and retractable seizures), or aspirin.

Nursing Interventions and Complications

Initial nursing management may begin in the critical care unit. The nurse vigilantly watches the basic human functions of respiration and cardiac/hemodynamic function. Small yet significant changes are assessed, monitored, and reported. Sudden patient deterioration can occur at any time.

The nurse monitors for hypoxia after head injury. The rationale for such continuous management includes decreased cardiac output, poor airway clearance, possible complication of associated chest trauma, aspiration status postinjury, or any other condition that impairs gas exchange.

It is possible that the patient is ventilated for added protection of the respiratory status. However, ventilation is applied judiciously and closely monitored because IICP can occur because of either vigorous suctioning or the overdistention of lung parenchyma dead space because of forced ventilation.

Invasive monitoring includes arterial lines that give accurate pressures. Measurement of core body temperature is required as deep brain damage can cause deficiency in thermoregulation. Arrhythmias are monitored via continuous ECG tracings and these can occur because of significant changes to body temperature, damage to certain areas of the brain that regulate heart rhythm, or electrolyte imbalances.

Hydration and nutrition are provided by artificial means via central lines or a peg tube. Because of the hypermetabolic state a patient with head injury may be in, enterally delivered nutrition provides the necessary nutrients needed to prevent negative protein balances that can contribute to acidosis. Careful fluid titration is monitored so as to not contribute to cerebral edema; therefore, fluids that are 5% dextrose are avoided. The patient will have an indwelling catheter, and skin integrity is monitored. Repositioning and removal of pressure over sensitive bony prominences is the mainstay of good nursing care.

Blood glucose levels, when allowed to rise, produce glucotoxicity. A degree of lactic acidosis occurs and this may contribute to cerebral edema. Glucose levels are monitored closely, especially if the patient is being administered corticosteroids for inflammation and edema. An insulin sliding scale may be ordered. At times, an insulin pump or insulin infusion may be indicated.

Positioning is not only important for prevention of skin breakdown, but appropriate positioning reduces the risk of venous congestion demonstrated in jugular vein distention. This can contribute to IICP.

The nurse may administer sedatives that allow for sleep and rest. In addition, the administration of propofol might be indicated to help reduce the aggressive metabolic state resulting from head injuries.

The role of the nurse after the critical care setting continues to focus on respiration and cardiac status, patient safety, rehabilitation, eventual discharge, psychosocial assessment, and family involvement. Patient teaching encourages independence using assistive devices, seat belt use, and muscle/tendon strengthening. Nutritional counseling is indicated in conjunction with assessment of speech and swallowing abilities.

Upon discharge, the role of the nurse expands into the community. Home environment, caregiver roles, medications, safety, nutrition/hydration and physical/occupational therapy become the primary assessment. Caregiver fatigue is also closely monitored by visiting nurses, and a home health aide through a local agency may be recommended.

CLINICAL ALERT

Patient safety is paramount. Safety incorporates airway management, prevention of arrhythmias, hydration to prevent electrolyte imbalances, and assessment of the home environment. Caring for the multivariable complications that can occur in a patient with head injury can be overwhelming for the family, patient, and/or the primary caregiver. Caregiver fatigue is also closely assessed and respite programs are recommended.

Seizures

The brain functions by nerve impulses generated by the neurons and associated structures within the brain. Aberrant firing of electrical discharges is the basic premise for a group of disorders categorized as epilepsy or seizure disorders.

The electrical discharges within the brain are classified as brain waves: alpha, beta, theta, and delta.

Seizure etiology is varied. Common etiologies include tumors of the brain, infection (bacterial, fungal, viral), congenital malformations, gross metabolic disorders, trauma to the brain (head injury [traumatic and nontraumatic]), and at times, the etiology is unknown.

When seizure activity occurs, it is thought that any one of the two major adaptive functions is impaired. Either there is excessive focal activity that cannot be controlled or there is a reduced inhibition of these impulses inherent to the body's compensatory measures. The aberrant electrical discharges can at times progress if allowed to continue, causing local damage as well as damage to the cortical and thalamic brain areas. Further destruction can include the brainstem.

Seizures are measured using an EEG. As the electrical discharge permeates, diencephalocortical inhibitors are excited. This causes a disruption of the electrical wave producing the clonic portion of the seizure. If this inhibitor is ineffective, a tonic state permeates.

Seizures are classified as partial seizures (focal origin) or generalized seizures (without focal onset). Partial seizures include simple, complex, and secondary generalization seizures. Generalized seizures include tonic-clonic (grand mal) seizures, absence (petit mal) seizures, myoclonic, and atonic seizures.

Partial seizures generally begin in one section of the brain hemisphere. At times, they may spread to other parts of the brain, however rarely. Because they are so localized, loss of consciousness does not occur. If the abnormal neuron firing does spread to the other hemisphere of the brain, the activity is called complex partial seizures. At this juncture, the patient may lose consciousness.

Generalized seizures occur when both hemispheres are affected simultaneously. Because of involvement bilaterally, loss of consciousness is frequent. The patient may exhibit absence seizures or grand mal seizures (Figure 1–4).

Clinical manifestations are based on the type of seizure experienced by the patient.

Partial seizures: simple partial seizure (SPS) and complex seizure (CS).

- Motor area affected: gross motor movement (SPS)
- Sensory area affected: somatic changes, tingling, visual, auditory, olfactory, and gustatory changes. Oftentimes, this is a preseizure affect known as an aura (SPS).

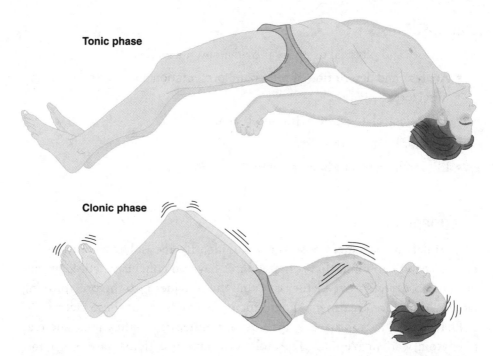

Tonic phase

Clonic phase

FIGURE 1–4 • Generalized tonic–clonic seizure, illustrating the appearance of the patient in the tonic (stiffening) and clonic (shaking) phases. (Reproduced with permission from Greenberg D, Aminoff M, Simon R, eds. *Clinical Neurology*. 8th ed. New York: McGraw-Hill; 2012, figure 12-2.)

- Loss of consciousness (CS)
- Automatisms: repetitive movements such as lip smacking, rubbing, and grimacing (CS)

Generalized seizures: absence seizure (AS), tonic-clonic seizure (TCS)

- Blank stares (AS)
- Unresponsiveness to verbal communication (AS)
- Automatisms (AS)
- Aura (TCS)
- Loss of consciousness (TCS)
- Incontinence—bladder and/or bowel (TCS)
- Tonic-clonic motor movements (TCS)
- Changes in respiratory rate (TCS)
- Postictal phase (TCS)

Diagnostic Tests

- History and physical exam by provider and nurse
- Analysis and description of preseizure presentation and post presentation of seizures activity
- Labs: electrolytes, CBC with differential
- MRI for brain abnormality
- EEG to help record brain activity

Treatment

The primary management of seizures is to identify and isolate a contributory factor. Keeping in mind that some seizures have no conclusive etiology, taking a full comprehensive history can clue the provider into the precipitating factors. Therefore, treatment should focus on avoidance of these factors.

Pharmacologic approaches include antiepileptic medications such as phenytoin, carbamazepine (Tegretol), ethosuximide, felbamate, tiagabine, levetiracetam (Keppra), lamotrigine (Lamictal), pregabalin (Lyrica), topiramate (Topamax), oxcarbazepine (Trileptal), or gabapentin (Neurontin).

Nursing Interventions and Complications

Nursing care is focused primarily on keeping the patient as safe as possible immediately before, during, and after a seizure. If the nurse suspects a seizure, gently guide the patient either to the bed, chair, or floor. Care should be taken in protecting the head, face, and limbs. Provide patient privacy because many patients fear behaviors during a seizure that might be embarrassing. Oftentimes, patients grab for blankets or other clothing items in an attempt to cover themselves.

Do not restrain the patient, and remain with the patient throughout the entire event. A calm, reassuring demeanor is necessary to avoid excess agitation of the patient. The nurse should promptly institute seizure precautions as necessary. An airway should be at the bedside in the event the respiratory tract becomes compromised. The nurse is reminded that other than an airway, nothing belongs in the mouth of the patient during a seizure.

Post seizure, vital signs are recorded. It is important to document the following as well: time of seizure, how long it lasted, were there any precipitating factors that prompted the event, did the patient have a change in behavior, or was there an aura. Note any incontinence. Note time of last seizure medication and promptly medicate if possible with next dose. At times, patients fall into a deep sleep post seizures; allow them to rest, constantly monitoring them.

CLINICAL ALERT

A major complication of seizures is status epilepticus.

Status epilepticus is a medical condition characterized by longer periods of seizure activity with shorter recovery periods. At some point, the seizures may become continuous without rest periods. If the patient has been seizing for 5 minutes or longer, status epilepticus is the medical diagnosis. This prolonged brain wave activity can occur because of being refractory to treatments, profound hypoglycemia, gross vitamin deficiencies, or alcohol withdrawal. The activity can either be convulsive or nonconvulsive but measurable on EEG.

During this prolonged period of seizure activity, brain anoxia occurs. The outcomes of the interventions are to stop the seizure activity and restore homeostasis.

Nursing management of the patient in status epilepticus occurs within a critical care setting. The following are the collaborative interventions for a patient exhibiting nonrelenting, prolonged seizure activity according to the U.S. Department of Health and Human Services, Agency for Healthcare Research and Quality, National Clearinghouse management of status epilepticus.

- *Airway assessment, preparing the patient for possible mechanical ventilation*
- *Medication administration: glucose (if seizure is due to profound hypoglycemia), thiamine (if due to prolonged deficiency), and agents to stop the seizures such as benzodiazepines, phenytoin, diazepam, lorazepam*
- *Vital signs assessment*
- *Continuous cardiac monitoring*
- *Transfer to the intensive care unit*

Spinal Cord Injury

Similar to head injuries, the spinal cord can be injured via traumatic and non-traumatic events. Excessive forces that are over the threshold of distribution along the spinal cord places the cord at risk for multiple injuries because it cannot handle forces that exceed its capacity.

The spinal column houses delicate tissue, CNs, and sensory and motor pathways. If damage occurs along a motor pathway, the patient will exhibit loss of control of movements and may experience a complete dysfunction, resulting in paralysis (paraplegia or quadriplegia). If damage occurs along a sensory pathway, there is a profound loss of sensation, perception, touch, vibration, thermoregulation, and pain sensation.

With injuries that include hyperflexion/extension of the spinal column, extreme rotational injuries, spinal cord compression (as seen with a diving incident), and penetrating spinal cord injuries, these tissues can become severed, bruised, or damaged.

As with the compensatory measures of all body systems, inflammatory responses occur after spinal cord injury. Ischemia, bleeding, and swelling continue. At times, the spinal cord is so edematous that full assessment of function is not possible until the inflammatory process is reduced.

If there is an entire spinal cord transection, all sensation below the level of the injury would be lost. This includes motor, sensory, reflex activity, lack of thermoregulation, loss of touch, and sexual dysfunction. Central cord injuries involve the cortex of the spinal column where important nerve roots run through: cervical, thoracic, and lumbar nerves. There will be some degree of loss to incomplete loss of motor function, loss of pain sensation, and lack of thermoregulation.

Four specific spinal cord syndromes are identified: complete lesion (transection), central cord syndrome, anterior cord syndrome, and Brown-Sequard syndrome. Damage to the anterior portion of the spinal cord has similar effects as a transection injury; however, there is additional loss proprioception awareness (loss of the righting reflex), as well as positional and vibratory deficits. Brown-Sequard spinal injuries consist of injuries that occur only to one lateral side of the spinal cord. On the nondamaged side of the spinal cord, there is loss of pain sensation, lack of thermoregulation, and lack of awareness of light touch. On the affected side, there is a profound loss of motor function, vibration, and positional sense.

Transection or complete lesions are devastating. High cervical transection can be fatal. Cervical injuries above C4 completely shut down the diaphragm's ability to function. The patient succumbs to respiratory dysfunction as intercostal muscles are also affected. If the patient survives, quadriplegia occurs. Loss of function in all four limbs in addition to the lower body is forever. C5 injuries are somewhat less devastating as innervation to muscles of the neck, shoulder and scapula is preserved. C6 injuries preserve most of the upper limb functions. C7 and C8 injuries preserve hand and wrist function.

Patients with high thoracic injuries can become paraplegic. To some degree, there may be some form of respiratory dysfunction but for the most part patients are able to breathe with minimal interventions. Upper motor and sensory pathways are preserved. From the waist down, they are immobilized. The extent of injuries along the thoracic region is directly dependent on the level of injury just like that in the cervical column. At T12, patients can regain some of their strength, ability, and flexibility with the use of assistive devices and intensive therapy.

Lumbar and sacral injuries preserve all of the upper extremities as well as almost all of the lower extremities. Patients with this level of spinal cord injury can walk after intensive therapy with minimal use of assistive devices.

Clinical Manifestations

Manifestations are based on the level of cord damage, the extent of cord damage, and the mechanism of injury.

Cervical injuries:

- Head and neck sequelae
- Diaphragm—respiratory distress
- Deltoids and biceps dysfunction
- Damage to the wrist
- Damage to the triceps
- Damage to the hand

Thoracic injuries:

- Diaphragm—respiratory compromise
- Damage to abdominal muscles—problems with gastrointestinal motility

Lumbar injuries:

- Leg muscles problems

Sacral injuries:

- Bowel and bladder dysfunction
- Sexual dysfunction

Diagnostic Tests

- X-ray
- MRI
- CT scan

Treatment

The damage caused from a spinal cord injury cannot always be reversed. Supportive treatment is indicated. As an immediate intervention, spinal cord stabilization after airway management is critical. Immobilization of the spine reduces the incidence of additional damage especially to sophisticated cervical and high thoracic discs.

Medications such as methylprednisone are given to help reduce spinal cord edema and evaluate loss of function. Traction may be indicated. A body harness or a halo (head traction) may be necessary. At times, a Philadelphia collar may be necessary to further stabilize the cervical column.

Surgical intervention may be required. Surgery is indicated when bone fragments or fractured discs compress the spine, and in the removal of foreign objects.

Nursing Interventions and Complications

In an emergent setting, the goal of the nurse is to maintain an airway and to stabilize the spine. Vital sign assessment implies continuous, vigilant monitoring for spinal shock. If the patient is aware, talking to the patient as diagnostics are completed, answering all questions from family members, and remaining at the patient's bedside are also very important. Nurses play a pivotal role in the early management of spinal cord injuries as the nurse is always with the patient in a critical care setting.

As spinal shock settles, the patient is further assessed. Daily range of motion, skin protection, turning, and repositioning are important. The nurse should also monitor for deep vein thrombosis secondary to inability to move. Management of bladder and bowel are also necessary as lower-level spinal cord injuries can cause impairment (neurogenic bladders), urinary stasis, increased risk for urinary tract infections, fecal impaction, and incontinence. The patient should be clothed properly because, oftentimes, thermoregulation is impaired.

Administration of medications, physical therapy consults, respiratory support, and nutrition are paramount. The patient may be eligible for extensive inpatient rehabilitation; therefore, the responsibilities of the nurse in this case may include pain management, use of supportive devices, bladder/bowel retraining programs, as well assisting the patient to be as independent as possible.

CLINICAL ALERT

Two significant complications of spinal cord injuries include spinal shock and autonomic dysreflexia.

When the spinal cord is shocked suddenly, its ability to adjust itself is impaired, especially if the injury is above T6. Spinal shock occurs after a sudden interruption of all neural pathways. The presence of shock is more pronounced with transection injuries. The nurse must monitor blood pressure as loss of parasympathetic systems produce profound hypotension. Heart rate and temperature monitoring are crucial because severe bradycardia may occur. Thermoregulation is problematic and patients usually lose their ability to sweat below the level of the injury.

Autonomic dysreflexia is an exaggerated response generated by the damaged spinal cord. Usually seen in patients with high spinal cord injuries, the patient exhibits very high blood pressures, headache, nasal congestion, restlessness, nausea, and blurred vision. Blood pressure can rise to 300 mm Hg systolic. This places the patient at risk for a stroke.

Nursing interventions require prompt awareness of spinal cord injuries and associated complications. Knowledge of the role of the sympathetic and parasympathetic responses and how these types of injuries can impair the pathways are important.

Vital sign assessment, early intervention, patient teaching, and prompt intervention are required.

Meningitis

The brain is surrounded by many protective layers. The outermost layer is the skull. Right beneath it are three layers that make up the meninges: the dura mater, arachnoid, and the pia mater (the layer closest to the brain parenchyma).

If these protective layers are compromised, pyogenic bacteria or viruses can enter the delicate brain tissues. At times, iatrogenic causes introduce these pyogenic agents.

When the microorganisms invade the meninges, meningitis occurs. Because cerebral spinal fluid is constantly circulating the brain and spinal column, the bacterial or viral agents quickly spread throughout the brain and spine. Bacteria of choice include *Escherichia coli*, *Neisseria meningitides*, *Streptococcus pneumonia*, and *Haemophilus influenza*. Viral agents include Human Papillomavirus and enteroviruses. Two other types of meningitis occur with fungal infections (cryptococcus or histoplasmosis exposure) and parasitic infections.

Gross inflammatory responses occur when there is infection. Edema and swelling of the delicate membranes occur. At times, the inflammation is so pronounced that circulation is impaired and necrosis develops.

Clinical Manifestations

- Malaise
- Fever
- Chills
- Headache
- Nuchal rigidity
- Light sensitivity
- Purpuric rash
- Positive Kerning sign
- Positive Brudzinski sign
- Seizures
- Drowsiness/lethargy
- Coma
- Death

Diagnostic Tests

- Lumbar tap (contraindicated of IICP) = high levels of protein, decreased glucose levels (spinal fluid analysis)
- Cultures of the spinal fluid and blood
- Chest x-ray
- CT scan of the head

Treatment
Nursing Interventions and Complications

The nurse should assess vital signs every 2 hours or more frequently as necessary. Neurologic assessments are completed as indicated, with prompt reporting of changes in neurologic status. This also includes assessment for seizures that can occur in a patient who has a fulminating infection or a parasitic infection. Keep a close eye on the level of consciousness. Pupillary changes indicate a deteriorating neurologic status. Patient comfort is maintained: repositioning, bathing, oral care, and provision of a quiet and calming environment. Medication administration (antibiotics, antipyretics, and antiinflammatory medications) are given and monitored for side effects, adverse effects, and therapeutic effects. Intake and output is measured. The nurse should also vigilantly monitor for Waterhouse-Friderichsen syndrome, a rare complication of bacterial meningitis.

CLINICAL ALERT

Monitoring for one of the most devastating complications of meningitis: Waterhouse-Friderichsen syndrome. Seen in fulminating meningitis, this complication can cause bacteremia/septicemia quickly. With this complication, the adrenal glands are also grossly affected. Adrenocortical necrosis can develop. The patient is assessed for high fevers, chills, backache, headache, and anorexia. Antibiotic treatment is early and aggressive because progression of the complication can lead quickly to loss of consciousness/coma and death.

Parkinson's Disease

Parkinson's disease is a disorder best explained as a disease of abnormal or alterations in movement. It is a common pathologic disorder seen in the older adult but has been noted in younger persons. The human body requires a balance between dopamine and acetylcholine (Ach). Dopamine is an inhibitory transmitter and it works synergistically with Ach, an excitatory transmitter that moves muscles. In Parkinson's disease, for reasons poorly understood, a degeneration of cells within the substantia nigra dies a slow yet progressive death. Lewy bodies, which are also seen in patients with dementia, are identified. With the loss of these cells, dopamine is depleted. In addition, other important neurotransmitters that are depleted include L-tyrosine hydroxylase, L-dopa-carboxylase, serotonin, and γ-aminobutyric acid (GABA). The coordinated depletion contributes to Parkinson's disease, but the most causative depletion is the dopamine neurotransmitter (Figure 1–5).

Clinical Manifestations

- Tremors (cardinal symptom)
- Rigidity (cardinal symptom)
- Bradykinesia (cardinal symptom)
- Loss of arm swing with walking

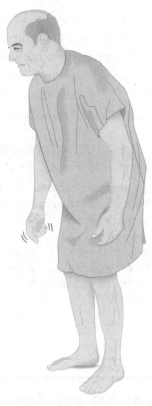

FIGURE 1–5 • Typical flexed posture of a patient with parkinsonism. (Reproduced with permission from Greenberg D, Aminoff M, Simon R, eds. *Clinical Neurology*. 8th ed. New York: McGraw-Hill; 2012, figure 11-4.)

- Monotone speech
- Small indecipherable writing
- Shuffling steps
- Spastic movements
- Akinesia
- Progressive loss of memory
- Dementia
- Loss of facial expression (masklike face)
- Inability to tolerate heat
- Bladder/bowel incontinence
- Depression
- Bradyphrenia

Diagnostic Tests

A complete neurologic examination is the cornerstone of diagnosis supported by additional radiographic tests. Symptomatology also aides in the diagnoses of Parkinson disease. Keeping in mind that there is no specific test for the diagnosis of Parkinson disease, MRI and CT scan can identify anatomic abnormalities although the brain of patients with Parkinson disease often appear normal. If there is an associated seizure disorder, an EEG is indicated.

Treatment

Treatments are centered around medications that improve symptoms. Carbidopa-levodopa crosses the blood-brain barrier. In the brain, the drug is converted to dopamine. The combination drug allows for carbidopa to protect the component of levodopa from premature conversion of the drug outside the brain.

Dopamine agonists such as pramipexole (Mirapex) and ropinirole (Requip) mirror the effects of dopamine within the brain. They usually have a longer mechanism of action, but fail to produce better symptom reduction of carbidopa-levodopa.

Patients may be started on coenzyme Q10 daily as it has demonstrated at slowing the incidence of motor deterioration. Monoamine oxidase B (MAO-B) inhibitors, noted to be effective adjuncts to therapy, help slow the progressive motor loss in Parkinson disease. These include rasagiline (Azilect) and selegiline (Eldepryl).

Recent studies are demonstrating effective results with deep brain stimulation. This modality is utilized in patients refractory to medications or in patients with poor response to levodopa. Deep brain stimulation helps reduce tremors and rigidity and improve overall symptoms. A small device is implanted within the chest wall cavity sending electrical impulses to the brain via implantable electrodes.

Nursing Interventions and Complications

Nursing interventions are centered on safety. Because of bradykinesia, freezing movements, uncoordinated gait, and tremors, the patient is at high risk for falls and injury. Medication administration as an inpatient and outpatient with appropriate education is critical. Some of the medications have significant side effects that include hallucinations. The patient should be assessed for depression, sexual dysfunction, psychosis, urinary dysfunction, and pain.

The nurse will need to discuss or encourage a discussion of end-of-life issues. Caregiver respite might be necessary as the disease has a long course. Challenges to transferring, positioning, walking/gait balance, and ADLs are important aspects for the nurse to address. Much of the care is in an outpatient environment; therefore, a visiting nurse may be recommended.

> ### CLINICAL ALERT
>
> *Prevention of further complications is a primary clinical alert. Use of assistive devices, removal of throw rugs, labeling of medications, follow-up appointments, and caregiver respite are all important alerts.*

Multiple Sclerosis

Multiple sclerosis is a neurodegenerative disease whose etiology is largely unknown. There might be an autoimmune component to the disease; it may be genetic in origin or can develop with the possibility of viral exposure. Nutritional habits, prolonged exposure to stress, and trauma have also been implicated.

In multiple sclerosis, changes to the white matter within the brain are seen. Plaque formation as well as degeneration of the myelin sheaths that cover the nerve endings occur. Destruction of the myelin sheaths prevents nerve transmission or impulses. When this occurs, the sensory, motor, cerebellar, visual, and bladder systems are affected.

Of the presenting symptoms, fatigue and visual changes occur. As the progressive destruction of the myelin sheaths persists, they become fibrotic (gliosis). It is thought that at times, some form of myelin sheath repair may occur, with resolution of some of symptoms; however, this is not the case at every presentation. In multiple sclerosis, the Schwann cells that are responsible for production of myelin are permanently destroyed (Figure 1–6).

There are four phases of multiple sclerosis:

- Progressive relapsing
- Secondary progressive
- Primary progressive
- Relapsing-remitting

An extremely rare presentation of multiple sclerosis is malignant multiple sclerosis or Marburg variant. This is an aggressive and progressive form of the disease that in a short period of time leaves the patient completely paralyzed.

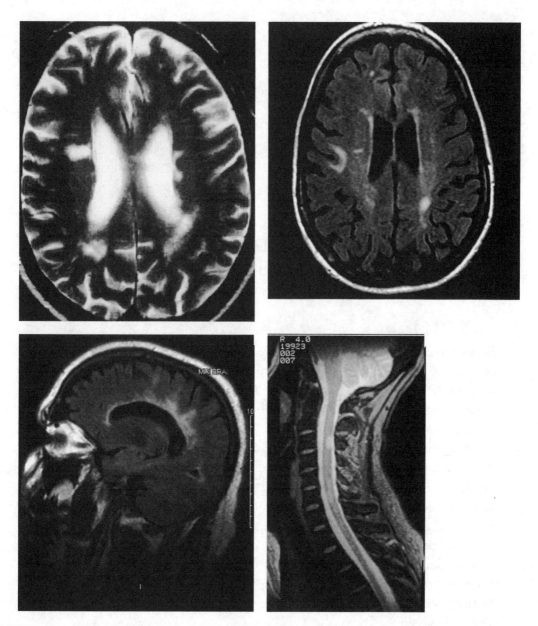

FIGURE 1–6 • Multiple sclerosis. T2-weighted and fluid-attenuated inversion recovery (FLAIR) sequence MRIs demonstrating multiple plaques in the periventricular white matter (*upper left*), emanating radially from the corpus callosum ("Dawson fingers"; *lower left*), a "C-like"–shaped lesion in the right subcortical white matter that is created by interruption of the lesion by the adjacent cortex (*upper right*), and cervical spinal cord (*lower right*). The radial orientation and periventricular location of cerebral lesions are typical of the disease. (Reproduced with permission from Ropper A, Adams M, eds. *Adams and Victor's Principles of Neurology*. 9th ed. New York: McGraw-Hill; 2009, figure 36-1.)

Clinical Manifestations

- Paresthesia
- Loss of proprioception
- Weakness
- Gait disturbance
- Fatigue
- Vision changes
- Nystagmus
- Bladder incontinence
- Changes in mood: depression, euphoria
- Cognitive dysfunction (in advanced disease)

Diagnostic Tests

Because the disease may wax and wane at presentation, prompt diagnosis is often difficult and lengthy. Oftentimes, patients go years suffering from symptoms frustrated that a diagnosis cannot be made. There are no single tests for the diagnosis of multiple sclerosis and symptomatology remains the central focus of diagnosis.

Additional tests may include MRI with gadolinium or a sophisticated MRI that measures brain parenchyma fracture (BPF), spinal lumbar tap (CSF assessment, myelin base protein), and evoked potential tests for muscle movement and brain activity if multiple sclerosis is suspected. For visual assessment, a visual evoked potential (VEP) may be indicated. A VEP is a test that measures the visual pathways to the brain.

According to the American Association of Neuroscience Nurses Multiple Sclerosis Practice Guidelines (2011), application of the Expanded Disability Status Scale (EDSS) can be used to help determine the extent of disability. The tool measures:

- Movement
- Coordination
- Visual perception
- Mental acuity
- Touch/pain

- Ability to maintain gait/balance/righting reflex
- Gag reflex
- Bladder/bowel functions

Treatment

Disease-modifying agents help reduce the exacerbations common to multiple sclerosis. They are also effective in reducing the number of plaques that build up within the brain parenchyma. Usually taken for long term, these medications significantly improve the quality of life among multiple sclerosis patients. A sample list of the medications include

- interferon beta-1a (Avonex or Rebif)
- interferon beta-1b (Betaseron or Extavia)
- glatiramer acetate (Copaxone)
- fingolimod (Gilenya)
- natalizumab (Tysabri)
- mitoxantrone (Novantrone)

Nursing Interventions and Complications

Disease-modifying agents are effective medications at controlling exacerbations but carry significant side effects that the nurse must monitor. Most are delivered via injection, so indurations at the injection site might be a problem. Other common side effects include flulike symptoms following injection. Anxiety, headache, lower respiratory tract infections, fatigue, bruising, alopecia, hair thinning, mouth sores, depression, chest pain, palpitations, shortness of breath, and flushing are other side effects that need to be monitored closely. The nurse teaches the patient to report the symptoms promptly.

CLINICAL ALERT

Bone marrow suppression is a real threat for the multiple sclerosis patient, especially if on Novantrone. Close monitoring of blood values, especially white blood cell counts as neutropenia, can complicate the course of treatment and put the patient at risk for infections given its ability to impair the immune system. In addition, liver function enzymes should be routinely monitored as Tysabri can cause significant liver dysfunction.

Guillain-Barré Syndrome

Guillain-Barré syndrome is another neurodegenerative disease that mimics multiple sclerosis in many ways. It is an acute polyneuritis. Both have no significant etiologic factors; however, a component of autoimmune destruction may play a part. It is believed that it can be triggered after exposure to an upper respiratory tract viral infection or a gastrointestinal infection. Although it is considered rare, it can present as an adverse effect of the influenza vaccine.

Once the disease presents, it is progressive, with symptoms evolving over hours, days, or even weeks. As with multiple sclerosis, there is a suggestion that an autoimmune response attacks the myelin sheaths of the nerves. Unlike multiple sclerosis, the Schwann cells are not destroyed; therefore, full recovery may be possible. However, 30% of patients are left with some residual weakness.

An IgM antimyelin antibody is responsible for the destruction of the myelin sheaths. The normal course of an inflammatory response brings lymphocytes and macrophages that contribute to the myelin destruction.

The body begins to regenerate its myelin sheaths and recovery can be slow or aggressive. Recovery can take days, weeks, to months. Body systems that lost their functional ability last regain function first.

Clinical Manifestations

- Bilateral lower extremity weakness
- Paresthesia of the lower extremities
- Progression of weakness to the upper extremities
- CNs are affected (all aspects of CN changes)
- Diaphragm paralysis (respiratory arrest)
- Facial paralysis
- If severe and aggressive, total paralysis requiring mechanical ventilation
- Bladder/bowel incontinence
- Pain, back and neck
- Loss of deep tendon reflexes
- Loss of gag reflex
- Diaphoresis
- Unstable vital signs

Diagnostic Tests

- CSF analysis
- Neurology assessment
- Deep tendon reflex analysis
- Nerve conduction velocity test

Treatment

There is no cure for Guillain-Barré syndrome; however, medications can manage the symptoms. Plasma exchange (plasmapheresis) to wash out the white blood cells from the blood can be undertaken. The red blood cells are returned to the patient. The rationale for the effectiveness of plasmapheresis is poorly understood; however, the removal of antibodies that destroy the myelin sheaths may be the answer. Corticosteroid therapy is often used to attempt to reduce the autoimmune inflammation but has not been proven to be of great help. High doses of immunoglobulin given intravenously have helped patients with Guillain-Barré syndrome.

Nursing Interventions and Complications

Because paralysis can occur rather rapidly, patients and families need emotional support. Verbalization of feelings is paramount. Patients who were once active on a daily basis are now dependent on others for ADLs and in some cases, if their respiratory status is challenged, are on mechanical ventilators.

Range of motion, skin protection, turning, and repositioning are important to prevent muscle atrophy, skin infections/breakdown, and the development of deep vein thrombosis.

Respiratory assessment should be ongoing as the disease may progress slowly or rapidly, and diaphragm paralysis is frightening for the patient.

CLINICAL ALERT

Monitor respiratory status continuously. Patients may require rehabilitation therapy, speech therapy, and psychological support. The nurse should be prepared to intervene as needed because of the psychological impact of the disease: paralysis.

CASE STUDY: NEUROLOGY

Dementia: Alzheimer Disease

The nurse is assigned a newly admitted 78-year-old female patient to the medical surgical/orthopedic floor. The patient was admitted through the emergency room after she fell at home earlier today.

Past medical history: hypertension (poorly controlled), hyperlipidemia, and dementia (Alzheimer, stage I)

Vital signs: BP (blood pressure) 148/98, HR (heart rate) 90, RR (respiratory rate) 20, temperature: 98.8°F

Patient is alert, mildly aggressive, knows her name and where she is, but cannot accurately place time and hour.

Medications: Enalapril 20 mg (QD), Zocor 20 mg (QD), Aspirin EC 81 mg (QD), Aricept 23 mg (QD)

Social history: Smoker × 30 years × 1 PPD (pack per day), quit 3 years ago, ETOH, daughter and son actively involved in patient care. Patient lives alone.

Upon assessment, the nurse asks questions determining safety, environment, nutrition, meals/meal planning, medications, and follow-up of appointments with providers. The patient is able to give her name, and inaccurately gave her home address and phone number. She can recall her daughter's and son's names and states that they don't visit often enough. She also appears to be having paranoid type of behaviors stating that someone keeps breaking into her home and stealing/misplacing her things constantly.

The daughter arrives to the unit and the nurse continues the inquiry asking similar questions to the daughter. She states that the patient has been getting more and more paranoid about her surroundings and that her apartment is littered with items she has picked up off the street. The daughter stated she found a rotten chicken in a pot inside the microwave today when she visited her mother's house to bring some of her personal effects to the hospital. The daughter also states that the police have been called to the apartment on numerous occasions with constant complaints of theft. The daughter is concerned over her mother's overall safety. She says that at first, she took her complaints of theft seriously but now worries that a cognitive change has occurred and that her dementia is now progressing. Up to this point, the patient has been able to live on her own although the daughter assumed all financial responsibility 3 months ago.

The nurse practitioner visits the patient and orders a right hip x-ray to rule out a fracture. Meanwhile, mild pain medications are ordered and given to keep the patient comfortable. The daughter remains at the bedside.

After the x-ray is reviewed, the determination is made that there is no hip fracture; however, a hematoma remains which is tender to palpation. The patient is kept overnight in preparation for discharge the next day. A referral to the social worker and a discharge planner as well as one for the visiting nurse service is completed by the attending nurse.

It is determined that the patient's overall cognitive status has decreased and that discharging her to home without supervision is unsafe. The daughter does not live close by and is unable to take the mother home to her house. It is decided that the patient will be more comprehensively assessed before discharge and a plan is set into place. Upon discharge, the patient will have 24 hour/7 day week home health aide supervision as determined by the hospital's home health agency. There will be weekly visits by the nurse who is responsible to monitor vital signs, assess nutritional status, and distribute medications. The nurse and the home health care agency will be in constant contact with the daughter, and the daughter has assured both that communication will be open and timely.

The following questions involve the overall presentation of a patient with Alzheimer. Use your critical thinking, your professional experiences, and the understanding of the pathophysiological changes that occur globally in the presence of Alzheimer disease to answer the following questions:

QUESTIONS

1. What were some of the clinical manifestations (objective and subjective) that sublimely gave indications that cognitive changes were occurring with this patient?
2. What are the three major safety considerations needed for this patient?
3. Is the planned discharge safe for this patient?
4. What would be important follow-up care for this patient?
5. What kinds of patient and family education are required for a safe discharge?

Suggested Readings

American Association of Neuroscience Nurses. *Nursing Management of the Patient With Multiple Sclerosis*. AANN, ARN, IOMSN Clinical Practice Guideline Series; 2011. http://www.rehabnurse.org/uploads/files/cpgms.pdf.

Gillick MR. Rethinking the role of tube feeding in patients with advanced dementia. *N Engl J Med*. 2000;342:206-210.

Habel M, VerHage A. Management of the patient with stroke. Nurse.com; 2011. http://ce.nurse.com/RetailCourseView.aspx?CourseNum=60074&page=2&IsA=1.

Helmy A, Carpenter KL, Menon DK, Pickard JD, Hutchison PJ. The cytokine response to human traumatic brain injury: temporal profiles and evidence for cerebral parenchyma production. *J Cereb Blood Flow Metab*. 2011;31:658-670.

Helmy A, Vizcaychipi M, Gupta AK. Traumatic brain injury: intensive care management. *Br J Anaesth*. 2007;99:32-42.

Ignatavicius D, Workman ML. *Medical-Surgical Nursing: Patient-Centered Collaborative Care*. 7th ed. St Louis, MO: Elsevier; 2013.

Maslow K, Mezez M. How to try this: recognition of dementia in hospitalized older adults. 2008;1:40-49.

Sharma A, Szeto K, Desilets AR. Efficacy and safety of deep brain stimulation as an adjunct to pharmacotherapy for the treatment of Parkinson's disease. *Ann Pharmacother*. 2012;46:248-254.

Stacy M, Davis TL, Heath S, Isaacson SH, Tarsy D, Williams M. The clinicians' and nurses' guide to Parkinson's disease. Medscape; 2009. http://www.medscape.org/viewarticle/701955.

Summers D, Leonard A, Wentworth D, et al. American Heart Association Council on Cardiovascular Nursing and the Stroke Council. Comprehensive overview of nursing and interdisciplinary care of the acute ischemic stroke patient: a scientific statement from the American Heart Association. *Stroke*. 2009;40:2911-2944.

Szaflarski JO, Rackley AY, Lindsell CJ, Szaflaski M, Yates SL. Seizure control in patients with epilepsy: the physician vs. medication factors. *BMC Health Serv Res*. 2008;8:264.

US Department of Health and Human Services, Agency for Healthcare Research and Quality. National Guideline Clearinghouse: EFNS guideline on the management of status epilepticus in adults. http://guideline.gov/content.aspx?id=24518, www.hhs.gov, www.ahrq.gov.

Yaffe K, Fox P, Newcomer R, Sands L, Dane K, Covinsky KE. Patient and caregiver characteristics and nursing home placement in patients with dementia. *J Am Med Assoc*. 2002;287:2090-2097.

Wehrle L. Epilepsy: its presentation and nursing management. *Nurs Times*. 2003;99:30-33. http://www.nursingtimes.net/epilepsy-its-presentation-and-nursing-management/205448.article.

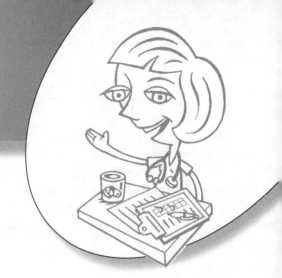

chapter 2

Respiratory System

LEARNING OBJECTIVES

At the end of this chapter, the reader/student will be able to:

● Describe the pathophysiology of the respiratory system components

● Compare the pathophysiology of pneumonia, tuberculosis, acute respiratory distress syndrome (ARDS), asthma, and chronic obstructive pulmonary disease

● Discuss and implement nursing measures in the management of respiratory disorders

Introduction

The respiratory system is a complex system that functions independently and codependently with multiple other systems. Beginning with the upper airway, which consists of the nose, oral cavity, and pharynx, the process of inspiration and expiration commences. The lower airway tract consists of the larynx, trachea, bronchi, and bronchioles with the eventual extension of the tract to the alveoli where actual gas exchange occurs. Both of the lungs consist of the apex (unlike the heart, this is the uppermost portion of the lung) and the base sitting right on top of the diaphragm. The right lobe consists of three lobes: the superior right lobe, the middle right lobe, and the inferior right lobe. The left lobe consists of two lobes: the superior left lobe and the inferior left lobe. Within the alveolar space, type I and type II cells support this structure. Type I cells consist of squamous epithelial cells and type II cells consists of surfactant-producing secretory cells that allow for lung expansion via allowance of surface tension. The final main portion of the respiratory system is the respiratory muscles. Inspiratory muscles consist of the diaphragm and are innervated by the phrenic nerve. Additional inspiratory muscles include the external intercostal muscles, the scalene muscle, and the sternocleidomastoid muscles. Expiratory muscles include the internal intercostal muscles and all the muscles along the abdominal wall structure.

Circulatory mechanisms are also complex. The lower and upper airways are supplied by bronchial circulation and pulmonary circulation. Bronchial circulation comes from the thoracic aorta, a dense bronchial arterial supply network and the upper intercostal arteries. The primary role of this circulatory pattern is to supply both lungs in its support of tissues, nerves, and multiple blood vessels. Pulmonary circulation is responsible for nurturing and maintaining perfusion through the alveolar-capillary membrane. Unlike system circulation, this pressure is lower, thus ensuring integrity of the delicate lung tissue. Lastly, the lymphatic drainage system plays a significant role within the respiratory system. Via the superficial and deep plexuses, drainage from the lungs and all of their supportive tissues and framework is effective and extensive.

The nerve supply to the respiratory tract extends from the brain and spinal column to include the first pair of cranial nerves: the olfactory nerve; the fifth pair of nerves: the trigeminal nerve; the seventh pair of nerves: the facial nerve; the ninth pair of nerves: the glossopharyngeal nerves; and the tenth pair of nerves: the vagus nerve. Nerves responsible for the larynx and pharynx include the eleventh pair of cranial nerves: the accessory nerves. Sympathetic and parasympathetic innervation controls the depth and breadth of the respiratory process.

Respirations occur through three active processes: the resting stage, the inspiration stage, and the expiration stage. During the resting stage, pressures outside and inside the pleural space are equal. The chest wall is relaxed and the diaphragm lies flat. During the inspiration stage, the chest wall moves out expanding and the diaphragm descends into the abdominal cavity. Intrapleural pressure becomes negative and intrapulmonic pressure becomes more negative, and the squeezing of the expansion of the chest wall increases pressure. During expiration, the chest wall moves inward, the diaphragm ascends, and intrapulmonic pressures become positive whereas intrapleural pressures remain negative. The cycle commences once again between always resting, inspiration, and expiration.

When the lungs are working as they should, breathing becomes effortless and proper oxygenation occurs. The lungs have extraordinary defense mechanisms that really work well in maintaining the integrity of the system. These defense mechanisms include the following:

- The mucociliary transport system
- The innate ability to ward off particulates within the airways
- Alveolar airway clearance
- Reflexes: gag reflex, sneeze reflex, and the cough reflex
- Hering-Breur reflex, which can be innately activated to prevent hyperinflation of the lung
- Immunologic defenses

Pneumonia

Pneumonia (PNA) is an inflammation of the lung structures: alveoli and bronchioles. These mechanisms are classified as: *typical* (bacteria, viruses, fungi [histoplasmosis, cryptococcus], nontubercular mycobacteria), *atypical* bacterial presentation, *hospital acquired (HAI)*, and *community acquired* pneumonia. Any disturbance or introduction of a foreign body into the lungs will manifest as an inflammation with subsequent inoculation of infection.

To better understand the pathogenesis of pneumonia, it is critical to be aware of the pathogens that bring on the disease process as it is common within communities and in health care institutions. Pneumonia development occurs as a result of exposure to virulent organisms, immunosuppression (cancer, radiation, chemotherapy, HIV), surgery, ventilator dependency, and immobilization, to mention a few. Proliferation of typical and atypical organisms can lead to different clinical manifestations and pathologic changes within the lung parenchyma.

Inappropriate or ineffective respiratory defense mechanisms also contribute to PNA development. Alterations in the glottic and cough reflexes that help protect against aspiration contribute significantly—especially in the presence of neuromuscular disease, stroke, abdominal or chest surgery, sedation, anesthesia, or with an obstruction such as a nasogastric tube. Dysfunction of the mucociliary tract due to a smoking history impairs the mobilization of secretions and micro-organisms along the respiratory tract. Finally, impairment of the immune system will also potentiate PNA. Changes in the phagocytic and macrophagic response due to smoking or immune-compromised states cannot produce an effective attack and remove offending micro-organisms.

Basic pathogenesis of PNA after insult sets off a cascading inflammatory response that is complex in nature. After infection, polymorphonuclear leukocytes (PMNs) along with monocytes and plasma proteins reach the affected alveoli. Neutrophils along with PMNs, proteins and monocytes accumulate within the alveoli. The monocytes after a few days mature into macrophages, beginning the process of bacterial destruction by engulfing the offending mechanism. The alveolar spaces are packed with the results of this inflammatory response. Blood leaks from the edematous capillaries, causing red hepatization that is seen as a discoloration of the lung tissue due to the results of the inflammatory process. Fibrin mesh deposits and erythrocytes after appearing days early into the infection turn gray in color, called gray hepatization. The lung is dense and friable, full of exudate. The end result is poor ventilation and pulmonary congestion. The infection tends to spread from lobe to lobe, segment to segment, through porous openings in the bronchial tree known as pores of Kohn. At the point of gray hepatization, the inflammatory response and medical intervention afford resolution of the infection.

Typical pneumonia: When bacterial, it is caused most commonly by the *Streptococcus pneumonia* (a gram-positive diplococcus). Exposure to this bacteria is the most common form of PNA and is typically also found with community-acquired PNA. Of the viruses, the bugs of choice are the rhinovirus and respiratory syncytial virus, bacterial *Haemophilus influenza*, and fungus *Pneumocystitis carinii*, coccidioidomycosis, histoplasmosis and cryptococcus (Figure 2-1).

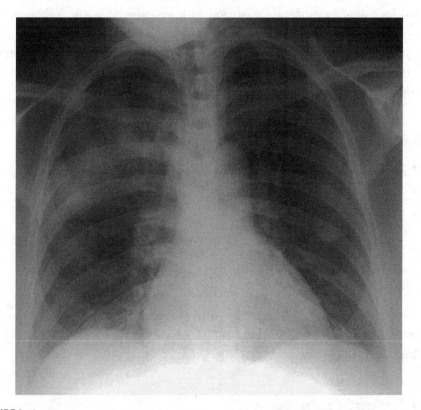

FIGURE 2–1 • Chest x-ray (CXR) showing right upper lobe consolidation. (Reproduced with permission from Miller WT Jr. *Diagnostic Thoracic Imaging*. New York: McGraw-Hill; 2006:218, figure 5-1B.)

Clinical Manifestations

- Cough
- Fatigue, generalized weakness, malaise
- Anorexia
- Fever (106.0°F), chills
- Pulmonary congestion—orthopnea, dyspnea, crackles, rhonchi
- Pleural friction/rub/pain
- Sputum production: red, green, rusty, yellow, yellow-green

Atypical pneumonia: What makes atypical PNA different from typical is the overall clinical presentation of this pneumonia. Different from typical PNA where the entire lung field is affected and spreading of the infection is common, atypical PNA is confined to the alveolar space with a lack of consolidation, small amounts of sputum production, and a low immunologic response manifested by a low or moderate elevation of leukocytes. It is also sporadic in its presentation, with significantly less mortality and morbidity rates than typical pneumonia. Its common bacterial causative factors are *Mycoplasma pneumonia*, *Chlamydia pneumonia*, or *H. influenza*. Viral atypical agents are adenovirus, rhinovirus, rubella, respiratory syncytial virus, and varicella.

Clinical Manifestations

- Fever
- Headache
- Muscle aches and pains
- Cough: dry, hacking, and nonproductive

Diagnostic Tests

The core of diagnostic testing for pneumonia includes sputum analysis and the chest radiograph. Additional diagnostics include the following:

- Arterial blood gases
- Pulse oximetry
- Fine-needle aspirations
- Pulmonary function tests

- Magnetic resonance imaging
- Computed tomographic scan

Treatment

Treatments are based on the type of pneumonia the patient presents with. The nurse must keep in mind that pneumonias as mentioned earlier are typical and atypical, and hospital or community acquired.

In caring for patients with community-acquired pneumonias, the nurse must remember that treating the patient as well as the family and providing education about the patient's surrounding environment are important. Patients should be taught to wash their hands and cover their nose and mouth when sneezing. Explain that respiratory particles can aerate 180 degrees and 3 feet forward. Patients also must be instructed to finish their antibiotics and take antipyretics for fevers as indicated.

Hospitalized patients require the basics of hygiene, clean environments, intact open portals of entry, redressing of wounds and lines, and timely administration of antibiotics and antipyretics. For both pneumonias, principles of pulmonary toileting are warranted.

Nursing Interventions and Complications

Pneumonia complications can extend from difficulty breathing to systemic infection. Respiratory insufficiency and respiratory arrest, though unlikely when nursing interventions are prompt, complicate the very old and the very young and anyone else that might be immunocompromised due to illness or medications, or are patients of organ transplants.

CLINICAL ALERT

Prompt assessments by the nurse are crucial in the management and prevention of complications of a patient with pneumonia. The nurse must monitor vital signs, respiratory rate, and respiratory function as well as oxygen saturation markers. Prompt administration of medications is an important intervention. Early mobility, pulmonary toileting, and use of the incentive spirometry are other significant nursing interventions that prove their weight in gold in managing and/or preventing pneumonia.

Tuberculosis

Pulmonary tuberculosis (TB) has been in existence for a very long time. Excavated mummies from Egypt have been found to harbor the dead bacterium known as *Mycobacterium tuberculosis*. This bacterium is a rod-shaped, aerobic, acid-fast bacillus that is spread through aerosolized droplets released through talking, coughing, sneezing, laughing, and singing. After successful intrusion of the infection chain through a portal of entry, the bacterium gains access to the airways and begins to grow and proliferate within its new host. If the patient has an intact immune system, the infection can lay dormant and inactive, never demonstrating signs and symptoms. If the infection occurs in a patient without an intact immune system, infection proliferates rapidly.

TB is common among foreign-born persons because of the higher risk for infection due to a high incidence rate and it is also prevalent in communities where large numbers of persons aggregate. Examples include the incarcerated, among the homeless population, and those who reside in shelters or any living situation that involves overcrowding.

Tuberculosis can be either primary or secondary. In primary disease, the host has had no previous exposure to *M. tuberculosis*. These patients harbor the bacilli; their bodies encapsulate the organism via T lymphocytes and macrophages developing latent TB. The encapsulated aggregation of macrophages infected with the bacillus is contained within the Ghon focus or complex. Often these are asymptomatic and never develop full-blown disease. Usually these patients have an intact immune system. They cannot pass the disease to anyone. Secondary TB occurs when the body is either reinfected or there is a reactivation of the disease. When impairment of the intact immune system occurs, it opens the door for activation or reinfection.

Clinical Manifestations (Secondary Infection Symptoms)

- Low-grade body temperature
- Fatigue
- Weight loss
- Night sweating/diaphoresis
- Nonproductive cough that later on becomes productive
- Blood-streaked sputum
- Positive skin test

- Anorexia
- Dyspnea later in disease progression
- Rales/rhonchi on lung auscultation

Diagnostic Tests

- Mantoux testing: intradermal injection of tuberculin
- Sputum analysis, but is not definitive for infection
- Chest x-ray: assessment of radiographic cavitations (Ghon complex) and/ or pleural effusions
- Three positive consecutive early morning sputum analysis
- Fiber optic bronchoscopy: assessment of bronchial washings, aspirate
- Needle biopsy of the pleural space

Treatment

Because of the ability of the tubercle bacillus to mutate at a high rate and its high ability to become resistant to one drug, drug combinations are utilized. New combination drugs are being developed in order to combat drug-resistant bacilli. However, the combination of medication that still holds a positive arsenal against TB includes isoniazid (INH), ethambutol, pyrazinamide, and rifampin. Treatment is reserved for those known to have active disease and for those who care for patients with active disease.

Nursing Interventions and Complications

The nurse must remain vigilant in his or her understanding of patients who are at risk for the acquisition and eventual clinical disease state of tuberculosis. At-risk patients include the following:

- Family members who are caring for a patient with TB
- Those who are already immunocompromised: HIV patients, cancer patients receiving chemotherapy/radiation and patients with organ transplants receiving antirejection medications
- The homeless
- Patients who abuse drugs and alcohol
- High-risk cohorts: those in correctional facilities, shelters, and health care workers

- Recent migration to the United States
- Medical risk factors also include diabetes mellitus (DM), chronic renal failure (CRF), leukemia, and those with medical conditions such as chronic obstructive pulmonary disease (COPD) that require long-term use of corticosteroids

Nurses must also assess patients and determine who should be routinely tested for TB. Routine testing of patients with low risk are not recommended. Keep in mind that testing does not distinguish between active or latent disease. Also, determine the patient's country of birth because exposure to the Bacille Calmette-Guérin (BCG) vaccine can cause a false-positive TB Mantoux test. If the patient is immunocompromised, false-negative tests can be produced, known as anergy, because the patient is unable to mount a response to the test or because he or she is not or has not been exposed to the bacilli.

Complications arise because of the length of treatment time. This encompasses lack of compliancy with medication regime. The Centers for Disease Control and Prevention in Washington, D.C., recommends directly observed therapy, short course (DOTS), management of the patient with TB who may not be compliant and pose a health risk for infecting others. Additionally, patients can develop drug-resistant TB if the regimen is not followed closely. Persons with concomitant infections of TB and HIV require close monitoring.

CLINICAL ALERT

- *Assessment of patients considered high risk*
- *Implementation of basic hygiene: hand washing, covering mouth when coughing*
- *Implementation of medication, often in combination*
- *Monitoring drug compliancy*
- *Monitoring follow-up therapy*

Pneumothorax

Within the tight walls of the pleural cavity, there is little room for anything other than the delicate balance between fluid, air, and tissue. However, because of various reasons, air can accumulate with the pleural cavity. Common etiologies for the accumulation of fluid include lung injury and trauma, but it can sometimes occur for no apparent reason. Pneumothoraxes are classified as either spontaneous or nonspontaneous. A small bleb or bulla can rupture and precipitate a pneumothorax. Lung collapse can be a common complication, and it can either be partial or complete. This is due to the pressure shifts that develop once air is introduced into the pleural space. Atmospheric air enters the airways upon bleb/bulla rupture and because the pressures within the alveolar pathways are greater than pleural pressures air will flow from the alveoli into the pleural space causing the lung collapse.

Clinical Manifestations

- Dyspnea
- Asymmetrical chest expansion
- Acute onset of ipsilateral chest pain
- Acute onset of shortness of breath
- Decreased tactile fremitus
- Diminished breath sounds
- Cyanosis
- Hypotension
- Unilateral chest expansion
- Hyperresonance over the lung field
- Tachypnea
- Changes in vital signs: mild tachycardia
- Mediastinal shift

Diagnostic Tests

- Blood work: arterial blood gases indicating hypoxemia and acute respiratory alkalosis
- Electrocardiogram: changes due to shifting mediastinal changes to the QRS complex and to the T wave
- Chest x-ray

Treatment

Supplemental oxygen is the treatment of choice. Usually, the excess amount of air is reabsorbed. When the pneumothorax is large, aspiration of the air by needles or closed system drainage is utilized.

Nursing Interventions and Complications

Vigilance for respiratory impairment is an important assessment by the nurse. Hypoxemia can occur quickly. This hypoxemia can be more adverse in patients with already complicated lung disorders or those who have a history of smoking.

Monitoring of oxygen saturation and for signs and symptoms of hypoxemia are critical. If the patient has a closed drainage system, proper maintenance and assessment of the system as well as skin integrity at the site of entry are important. Advise the patient that frequent chest x-rays might be necessary to determine how much air is left in the pleural cavity. Allay fears of exposure to radiation and explain the risks and benefits of diagnostics.

> ### CLINICAL ALERT
>
> *Monitor oxygen saturation closely. Assessment of any changes to the respiratory status is important, and prompt reporting is essential. Ensure that the patient receives the correct amount of oxygen with the correct mode of application. Auscultate lung sounds often. Assess for any hyperactivity, disorientation, and confusion especially among the elderly as these may be primary indicators of drops in oxygen saturation.*

Acute Respiratory Distress Syndrome (ARDS)

Introduction

ARDS is an inflammatory response to acute lung injury. Etiology for lung injury can include several conditions: lung infections or bacteremia, when a patient suffers trauma (burns), a fat embolism, near-drowning situations, drug intoxification, smoke inhalation injuries, or as a result of diffuse coagulopathy such as disseminated intravascular coagulation. Injury can be categorized as direct or indirect epithelial lung damage. Synergistically, aside from ARDS, acute lung injury (ALI) is a less intense response to lung injury that, if not aggressively assessed and managed, can advance to ARDS.

Epithelial cell injury occurs and as this injury transitions, there is increased permeability across the alveolar-capillary cell membrane. Increasing amounts of fluid, proteins, and blood moves into the tight alveolar spaces altering gas exchange. The patient begins to have a great deal of difficulty breathing, gas exchange diminishes, hypoxemia ensues, and the lung, because it is injured, becomes less pliant and more susceptible to damage. Surfactant, the substance that keeps the alveoli open, is inactivated, further complicating the process. Despite high levels of oxygen administration, the ARDS patient still struggles to breathe, and tissues continue to lack oxygen. Although the exact mechanisms are unknown as to how the lung responds to the injuries noted above, a gross inflammatory process at both the local and systemic level appears to trigger ARDS. Keep in mind that whenever there is injury or inflammation, neutrophils are activated. In ARDS, neutrophil activation causes congestion because it tends to secrete enzymes and phospholipid products that can further add to the inflammatory response. Over time, the body can reabsorb all the debris accumulated from the inflammatory response; however, the patient may require ventilatory support during this transitional phase.

Clinical Manifestations

- Rapid and progressive shortness of breath (12–18 hours)
- Changes to respiratory pattern: tachypnea, use of accessory muscles, retracted breathing, labored in nature, moist rhonchi/rales auscultated
- Hypoxemia
- Multiorgan failure
- Changes in chest x-ray

Diagnostic Tests

- Chest x-ray
- Oxygen saturation

Treatment

If hypoxemia continues, patients often are refractory to supplemental oxygen. Ventilatory support is therefore indicated. High-flow oxygen is administered. The goal is to profuse the supportive body systems and allow the lungs time to heal and retract from the acute inflammatory response. Positive end-expiratory pressures (PEEPs) are often applied to assist the alveoli reinflate.

Nursing Interventions and Complications

- Assess for patients at risk for the development of ARDS: septicemia, pancreatitis, disseminated intravascular coagulation (DIC), head trauma, thrombus embolism, TB, near-drowning victims, aspiration of gastric contents

- Manage ventilated patient: infection control, skin integrity, mobility, nutrition, hydration, weaning from ventilator, treatment of any wounds
- Complications include ventilator-induced pulmonary infections: monitor vital signs, assess for sign or symptoms of respiratory difficulty, apply suction per protocol

---

CLINICAL ALERT

Assessment of patients who, because of possible lung injuries, might progress to ARDS. Determine the ALI of the patient and anticipate possible changes to his or her respiratory status. ARDS can lead very quickly to acute hypoxemic respiratory failure. Monitor ventilation-perfusion ratios (VQ), because a change or a mismatch in VQ perfusion is an indicator of respiratory problems.

Asthma Introduction

Asthma falls under the category of obstructive airway disorders. Similar to chronic obstructive airway disease, bronchial constriction limits airway movement. Unlike chronic obstructive airway disease, asthma is reversible and is often an acute process. Parasympathetic and sympathetic mechanisms work synergistically, controlling air movement. The vagus nerve is stimulated by cholinergic receptors, thus producing bronchoconstriction. Sympathetic responses occur through β_2-adrenergic receptors causing bronchodilation. When the body needs increased oxygenation, such as with exercise or in times of stress, the sympathetic nervous system kicks in. This normal process is altered when an inflammatory response occurs within the bronchus. Wheezing, difficulty breathing, and chest tightness are triggered when the person is exposed to allergens that set off the inflammatory response. A hypersensitive response ensues. An influx of white blood cells (a common response in inflammatory processes) and mast cells eventually clutter and damage the bronchus. When this occurs, a restrictive process occurs. Chronic exposure causes remodeling of the epithelial lining of the bronchus. Airflow is limited, and edema and continued epithelial injury persists, as well as an impairment of the mucociliary functions that are designed to move secretions. This leads to increased airway responsiveness, or asthma.

There are two types of asthma. Extrinsic asthma occurs in response to an antigen and is considered a type I hypersensitivity. Intrinsic asthma is a respiratory response because of a nonimmune exposure. These include upper or lower respiratory tract infections, exercise, stress or exposure to bronchial irritants such as occupational exposure, direct or secondhand cigarette/tobacco smoke exposure.

Additionally, a subgroup of patients with asthma falls under the category of severe asthma. Often for unknown reasons or perhaps because of a genetic component to the hypersensitive asthmatic response, this small yet significantly important category of patients may have fatal or near-fatal asthmatic responses. Oftentimes, it is the underestimation of how acute a previous flare-up was that places these patients at risk because they may delay in seeking treatment that can be life-saving.

Asthmatic severity can be categorized as follows:

- **Mild intermittent:** symptoms are present less than 2 days/week and there is no interference with activities of daily living (ADLs), good medication response to short-acting β_2-agonists, forced expiratory volume in 1 second (FEV$_1$) >80% predicted.

- **Mild persistent:** symptoms are present at least 2 days a week but not every day and there is some degree of interference with ADLs, good medication response to short-acting β_2-agonists (however, patient begins to use the medication more and more), and FEV$_1$ is >80% predicted.

- **Moderate persistent:** symptoms occur on a daily basis and continued interference with ADLs continue, medication response to short-acting β_2-agonists begins to problematic and patient now uses the medication on a daily basis, FEV$_1$ <60% normal but <80% predicted.

- **Severe persistent:** symptoms are persistent every day and ADLs are not possible, medication response to short-acting β_2-agonists is now several times a day, FEV$_1$ <60% normal.

Clinical Manifestations Depend on Classification of Asthmatic Response

Mild attack:

- Chest tightness
- Elevated respiratory rate
- Anxiety

- Some wheezing
- Possible cough

Severe attack:

- Wheezing progresses
- Feelings of impending doom
- Chest tightness
- Marked anxiety
- Cough
- Fatigue
- Distant breath sounds
- Tachypnea
- Shortness of breath that is severe
- Use of accessory muscles
- Limited ability to speak

Impending respiratory failure:

- Diminished breath sounds (complete occlusion of bronchus)
- Fatigue
- Diminished breath sounds
- Ineffective cough

Diagnostic Tests

- Classification of asthma severity assessment

Pulmonary function test (PFT): spirometry. The measurement of the FEV_1 is critical to assessment in spirometry. FEV_1 is defined as the maximal volume that a patient can expire during a specific time frame starting from maximal inspiration. The subscript indicates time in seconds. An FEV_1 greater that 80% is normal, an FEV_1 of 60%–79% indicates mild airway obstruction, an FEV_1 of 40%–59% indicates moderate obstruction, and an FEV_1 of below 40% indicates severe airway obstruction.

- Arterial blood gases
- Peak expiratory flow meters
- Chest x-ray
- Skin testing to rule allergens

Treatments

Medications to treat asthma depend on the severity of the attack.
Short-term medications include

- anticholinergic agents
- systemic steroids
- short-acting β_2-agonists

Long-term medications include

- inhaled steroids
- bronchodilators
- leukotriene pathway inhibitors
- theophylline
- cromolyn

A step down–step up approach to management of asthmatic symptoms is employed (Table 2–1).

Nursing Interventions and Complications

Patients should be taught to avoid allergens that are known triggers. These include respiratory infections, environmental triggers, exercise, changes in weather (humidity), irritants (perfumes, smoke), medications (nonsteroidal antiinflammatory drugs [NSAIDs], beta-blockers), and certain foods. Those who are not aware of triggers should visit an allergist. Patients should be taught to be more aware of their bodies and seek medical care when the use of short-acting β_2-agonists is increasing or when they are not getting a therapeutic response from their medications. Assess whether the patient has been previously hospitalized for an asthmatic attack. These patients will mostly have exaggerated responses in the future especially if they have been placed on ventilators because of respiratory failure.

CLINICAL ALERT

Teach patients to monitor and manage their symptoms using the step approach. It is important that they are aware of triggers and avoid them. Patients should follow up with influenza and pneumococcal vaccines. Patients should stop smoking and/or avoid smoke as it is a known trigger. Alert patients to seek prompt medical attention if they are not responding to their medications in a timely manner.

TABLE 2–1 Asthma Management—Youths ≥12 Years of Age & Adults (Part 1 of 2)

Classifying Asthma Severity and Initiating Treatment In Youths ≥12 Years of Age and Adults

Assessing severity and initiating treatment for patients who are not currently taking long-term control medications

Components of Severity		Classification of Asthma Severity (≥12 Years of Age)			
		Intermittent	Persistent		
			Mild	Moderate	Severe
Impairment Normal FEV_1/FVC: 8–19 yr 85% 20–39 yr 80% 40–59 yr 75% 60–80 yr 70%	Symptoms	≤2 days/week	>2 days/week but not daily	Daily	Throughout the day
	Nighttime awakenings	≤2×/month	3–4×/month	>1×/week but not nightly	Often 7×/week
	Short-acting β_2 agonist use for symptom control (not prevention of EIB)	≤2 days/week	>2 days/week but not daily and not more than 1 × on any day	Daily	Several times per day
	Interference with normal activity	None	Minor limitation	Some limitation	Extremely limited
	Lung function	• Normal FEV_1, between exacerbations • FEV_1 >80% predicted • FEV_1/FVC normal	• FEV_1 >80% predicted • FEV_1/FVC normal	• FEV_1 >60% but <80% predicted • FEV_1/FVC reduced 5%	• FEV_1 <60% predicted • FEV_1/FVC reduced >5%

Risk		0–1/year		≥2/year	
	Exacerbations requiring oral systemic corticosteroids	← Consider severity and interval since last exacerbation → Frequency and severity may fluctuate over time for patients in any severity category Relative annual risk of exacerbations may be related to FEV_1			
Recommended Step for Initiating Treatment		Step 1	Step 2	Step 3	Step 4 or 5 and consider short course of oral systemic corticosteroids
		In 2–6 weeks, evaluate level of asthma control that is achieved and adjust therapy accordingly.			

EIB, exercise-induced bronchospasm; FEV_1, forced expiratory volume in 1 second; FVC, forced vital capacity.

Adapted from National Asthma Education and Prevention Program. *Expert Panel Report 3: Guidelines for the Diagnosis and Management of Asthma 2007.*

U.S. Department of Health and Human Services. Available at http://www.nhlbi.nih.gov/guidelines/asthma/asthgdln.pdf. Accessed on: September 21, 2007.

Chronic Obstructive Pulmonary Disease (COPD)

Known as an obstructive airway disease, COPD interferes with the flow of air in and out of the lungs. In COPD, the obstruction is progressive and destructive. Under the umbrella of COPD are three main disorders: emphysema, chronic bronchitis, and bronchiectasis. In emphysema, there are changes to the airway space, usually an enlargement as air becomes trapped. In chronic bronchitis, there is hyperplasia of the bronchus and hypersecretion of the mucous glands, and in bronchiectasis, there is airway enlargement as well as remodeling or scarring of the bronchus. In emphysema and chronic bronchitis, the etiology is straightforward: smoking. Bronchiectasis with bronchial scarring occurs in persistent and frequent airway infections.

In COPD, airway irritation causes many ill effects on the airways.

When there is hypersensitivity and hyperreaction, the airways rather than the alveoli produce excessive amounts of secretion through the goblet cells of the airways. The basal cell membrane of the airways also becomes hyperplastic, remodeled by thickening. When there is inflammation, there is an aggregation of lymphocytes and macrophages. This congestion along with accumulating secretions causes airway obstruction. The airways eventually lose their integrity, closing prematurely during the expiration process. When this happens, air becomes trapped. Body systems do not work alone and all have some kind of interchangeable processes. In COPD, when the kidneys register low oxygen levels because of air trapping, it stimulates the production of erythropoietin to stimulate red blood cell formation. Remembering that red blood cells carry the oxygen molecule and the body is simply responding to low oxygen levels (hypoxia), thick blood develops. This factor in and of itself can interfere with blood circulation and the deliverance of oxygen.

Bronchitis—The Blue Bloater

In COPD, the chronic bronchitis patient is known as the blue bloater. These patients may demonstrate a degree of cor pulmonale (right-sided heart failure). Oftentimes, these patients are obese and have frequent cough with sputum production. They use their accessory muscles to breathe, have coarse rhonchi, and may wheeze. Their clinical presentation often mimics that of congestive heart failure. These patients progress in the dyspnea status, have frequent respiratory infections, and over time, can progress to either cardiac or respiratory failure. Edema and weight gain are common (Table 2–2).

TABLE 2–2 Classification of COPD by Severity (GOLD)	
Stage	**Characteristics**
0: At risk	Normal spirometry
	Chronic symptoms (cough, sputum production)
I: Mild	FEV$_1$/FVC <70%
	FEV$_1$ ≥80% predicted
	With or without chronic symptoms (cough, sputum production)
II: Moderate	FEV$_1$/FVC <70%
	30% ≤FEV$_1$ <80% predicted (11A: 50% ≤FEV$_1$ <80% predicted) (11B: 30% ≤FEV$_1$ <50% predicted)
	With or without chronic symptoms (cough, sputum production, dyspnea)
III: Severe	FEV$_1$/FVC <70%
	FEV$_1$ <30% predicted or FEV$_1$ <50% predicted plus respiratory failure[a] or clinical signs of right heart failure

[a]Respiratory failure = arterial partial pressure of oxygen (PaO$_2$) <8.0 kPa (60 mm Hg) with or without arterial partial pressure of CO$_2$ (PaCO$_2$) >6.7 kPa (50 mm Hg).
Reproduced with permission from Hanley M, Welsh C, eds. *Current Diagnosis & Treatment in Pulmonary Medicine.* New York: McGraw-Hill; 2003, table 7-1.

Clinical Manifestations

- Chronic nonrelenting cough that is productive
- Dyspnea (mild)
- Rhonchi
- Fever, chills
- Cyanosis
- Wheezing
- Significant drop in oxygen saturation
- Age 40–45

Diagnostic Tests

- PFTs
- Chest x-ray
- CT scan of the thorax
- Echocardiogram (to determine pulmonary hypertension)

Emphysema—The Pink Puffer

The patient with emphysema usually are the typical presenters of the barrel chest deformity common among COPD patients because of years of air trapping and rib cage widening to accommodate the persistent trapped air within. This is known as barrel chest. The normal diameters in a patient without COPD are as follows: anteroposterior diameter/transverse diameter = 1/2. In COPD, the AP diameter/transverse diameter = 2. Unlike the chronic bronchitis patients, their cough is little to almost none, with no sputum production. Purse lipped breathing aids with air/gas exchange. Breathing in a sitting upright position is easiest for these patients as they use their accessory muscles to breathe. Heart sounds are distant, and wheezing may be present. The emphysemic patient has a long history of smoking, progressive cough and dyspnea, weight loss, and eventual respiratory failure.

Clinical Manifestations

- Severe dyspnea
- Cough (although rare)
- Weight loss
- Use of accessory muscles
- Rare drop in oxygen saturation

Diagnostic Tests

- PFTs
- Chest x-ray
- CT scan of the thorax
- Echocardiogram (to determine pulmonary hypertension)

Treatment

Treatment for both emphysema and chronic bronchitis centers on the common goal of oxygenation, management of symptoms, smoking cessation, and quality of life. Depending on the stage of the COPD, treatment requires a multidisciplinary approach. Smoking cessation is a priority. Every effort should be made to encourage smoking cessation by setting a stop goal date and supportive measures to include medications as well as attending a smoking cessation counselor/session. The patient should be encouraged to remain as active as possible, attend pulmonary rehabilitation programs, and complete breathing exercises. Prompt management of respiratory tract infections are critical to prevent deterioration of the already oxygen-compromised patient. Vaccination with the influenza vaccine annually and the pneumonia vaccine are also important and should be stressed by the nurse.

Medications include bronchodilators and inhaled adrenergic and anticholinergic agents. These drugs work by inducing bronchodilation and reducing sputum volume. Oral theophylline and steroids are other effective medications. Oxygen therapy is a mainstay for the COPD patient but caution must be exercised in limiting the flow of oxygen to no more than 2 L/minute. Goal of oxygen therapy is to maintain an O_2 saturation of at least 90%.

Nursing Interventions and Complications

When assessing the patient for COPD, it is important to keep in mind the risk factors of the disease. They include smoking cigarettes, inhalation of second-hand smoke, being of a low socioeconomic status, being non-Caucasian and male, exposure to occupational air pollution, having hyperactive airways, and α_1-antitrypsin deficiency (a genetic trait that causes damage to the lungs and liver). Ensure that patients take their medications. Caution when giving oxygen at levels above 2 L/minute remembering that the respiratory drive can be suppressed because of high levels of oxygen. Monitor patient for the following complications and be prepared to intervene appropriately:

- Respiratory distress/failure/arrest
- Right-sided heart failure (cor pulmonale)
- Pulmonary hypertension
- Pneumothorax
- Hemoptysis
- Pneumonia
- Pulmonary embolism

CLINICAL ALERT

The most important clinical alert with COPD is the amount of oxygen delivered, smoking cessation, and the prompt identification and management of respiratory infections. These states can significantly hamper the overall prognosis of COPD patients as their respiratory status is already compromised. Enforcing smoking cessation, taking antibiotics when sick, and vaccination are also paramount.

CASE STUDY: RESPIRATORY

Pneumonia

Mrs. LG, an African American, comes to the provider's office with multiple general complaints. She informs the nurse doing the intake that she has been coughing for about 3 days with very little sputum production. She states that she feels as though she had a fever and some accompanying chills, but that they only lasted for 1 day. She feels fatigued, malaise, anorexic, and weak. Mrs. LG reveals that she just cannot find the strength to get out of bed and if it had not been for the insistence of her husband to come to the provider's office today, she would have much rather stayed in bed at home.

The nurse reviews the patient's chart:

PMH (pure motor hemiparesis): cerebrovascular accident (CVA) with left-sided weakness, 2004; TIA (transient ischemic attack) × 2, 2005 and 2010, both of which left additional weakness on the left side. Lobectomy right breast 2012, hyperlipidemia, and hypertension. The patient also had a strong smoking history, although she stopped smoking about 20 years ago.

Medications: Xanax 0.5 mg (BID) PRN (as needed) for mild anxiety, Lexapro 10 mg (QD) for depression, Micardis 80 mg (switched from an ACE [angiotensin-converting enzyme] inhibitor because of cough), and Livalo 4 mg (QD).

Vital signs: BP (blood pressure) 138/88, HR (heart rate) 109 and although tachycardic, is of regular rhythm, RR (respiratory rate) 26, temperature: 99.0°F

The nurse inquires about medication history and the patient confirms that she has been taking her medications as ordered with the assistance of her husband, who is her primary caregiver.

Upon lung auscultation, there are significant adventitious breath sounds heard and a question about a possible pleural rub. The rub can be auscultated over the left lung and is significantly audible. The patient states that taking a deep breath hurts her. The husband seems surprised by her statement and proceeds to ask her why she did not tell him before that she was in pain.

The provider orders a stat chest x-ray, and a left lower lobe consolidation is seen on radiograph. The patient is duly admitted to the hospital for treatment of pneumonia, fatigue, and possible dehydration, given her elevated heart rate and temperature, as well as the fact that she has not eaten or had fluids over the last few days.

The nurse admits the patient to the respiratory unit after initial assessment in the emergency department. The following questions are in regard to the expected care and nursing interventions of this patient.

Suggested Readings

Blancherette CM, Berry SR, Lane SJ. Advances in chronic obstructive pulmonary disease among older adults. *Curr Opin Pulmon Med*. 2011;17:84-89.

Bloss E, Chan P-C, Cheng N-W, Wang K-F, Yang S-L, Cegielski P. Increasing directly observed therapy related to improved tuberculosis treatment outcomes in Taiwan. *Int J Tuberc Lung Dis*. 2012;16:462-467.

Ignatavicius D, Workman ML. *Medical-Surgical Nursing: Patient-Centered Collaborative Care*. 7th ed. St Louis, MO: Elsevier; 2013.

Eisner MD, Parsons P, Matthay MA, Ware L, Greene K. Acute respiratory distress syndrome network. Plasma surfactant protein levels and clinical outcomes in patients with acute lung injury. *Thorax*. 2003;58:983-988.

Matthay MA, Zimmerman GA. Acute lung injury and acute respiratory distress syndrome: four decades of inquiry into pathogenesis and rational management. *Am J Respir Cell Mol Biol*. 2005;33:319-327.

National Lung, Heart, Blood Institute National Asthma Education and Prevention Program. *Expert Panel Report 3: Guidelines for Diagnosis and Management of Asthma*. Bethesda, MD: National Institutes of Health; 2007.

Noppen M. Spontaneous pneumothorax: epidemiology pathophysiology and cause. *Eur Respir Rev*. 2010;19(117):217-219.

Stone IS, Barnes NC, Petersen SE. Chronic obstructive pulmonary disease: a modifiable risk factor for cardiovascular disease? *Heart*. 2012;98:1055-1062.

Sveum R, Bergstrom J, Brottman G, et al. Institute for Clinical Systems Improvement. Diagnosis and Management of Asthma. http://bit.ly/Asthma0712. Updated July 2012.

Willis MD, Winston CA, Heilig CM, Cain KP, Walter ND, Mac Kenzie WR. Seasonality of tuberculosis in the United States, 1993-2008. *Clin Infect Dis*. 2012;54:1553-1560.

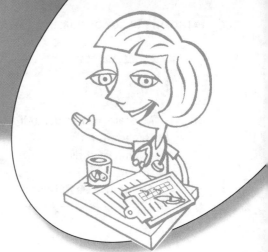

Cardiovascular System

LEARNING OBJECTIVES

At the end of this chapter, the reader/student will be able to:

● Describe the pathophysiology of major cardiovascular system components

● Compare the pathophysiology of myocardial infarctions, hypertension, angina pectoris, atherosclerosis, heart failure (right and left heart), rheumatoid fever, and valvular disorders

● Discuss and implement nursing measures in the management of cardiovascular disorders

KEY WORDS

Myocardial Infarction (MI)
Hypertension
Angina Pectoris
Atherosclerosis
Congestive Heart Failure

Rheumatic Fever
Valvular Disorders
Mitral Valve Disorders
Aortic Valve Disorders

Introduction

The cardiovascular system consists of the main organ, the heart, the incorporation of the respiratory system for oxygenation, and a complicated and extensive network of blood vessels, lymphatic vessels, metabolic pathways, and millions of cells that produce the effect of the pumping action and the electrical action of the heart.

The heart is composed of three main layers: the epicardium, which is a thin, transparent outer layer consisting of the mesothelium and connective tissue; the myocardium, which is the middle layer consisting of cardiac muscle fibers that are striated and branched, operating under involuntary control; and the endocardium consisting of a thin layer of endothelium overlying more connective tissue. Surrounding and protecting the heart is a triple layer of fibrous pericardium and serous pericardium tissue. This is called the pericardium.

The heart consists of four chambers: the two atrias and the two ventricles. Each supports the heart in its continuous role to supply blood and oxygen to all body tissues. In addition, there are four major heart valves that help move blood throughout the heart: the atrioventricular valves, consisting of the tricuspid valve and the mitral valve, and the semilunar valves, which are made of the pulmonic valve and the aortic valve. These valves play an important role in moving blood through the heart, preventing regurgitation, and respond to pressure changes within the heart. The audible heart sounds consist of the opening and closing of the cardiac valves. The first sound (S_1) is louder and longer than the second heart sound (S_2). The S_1 sound occurs as turbulent blood flows through the tricuspid and mitral valves and they close in response to pressure changes due to varying blood volume. The second heart sound (S_2) is heard as the pulmonic and aortic valves close.

The flow of blood through the heart is an easy concept to visualize. Deoxygenated blood (blue blood) enters the heart from the body system via the superior and inferior vena cava. Blood enters the right atrium through the tricuspid valve into the right ventricle. The ventricle contracts in response to pressure changes caused by increased volume and heart stretch (Starling law) pushing blood through the pulmonic valve into the pulmonic trunk that bifurcates into the right and left pulmonary artery. Once in the lungs, gas exchange occurs at the alveolar level. Oxygen transport (red blood) occurs and the blood is then pushed back through the right and left pulmonary veins into the left atrium, through the mitral valve into the left ventricle (the largest and most powerful portion of the heart) and then up and out through the aortic valve into systemic circulation. This process occurs hundreds of thousands of time in a person's lifetime.

Blood cannot move through the heart without electrical current. Cardiac cells are energized because of the rudimentary development of autorhythmic (self-excitable) cells that develop during the embryonic stages. These autorhythmic cells act as the heart's pacemaker, helping it beat in a pattern conducive to blood movement, and they also serve as cells that are part of the conduction system. Within the conduction system that these cells innervate are important internal pacemakers: the sinoatrial (SA) node, the atrioventricular (AV) node, the AV bundle, also known as the Bundle of His, the right and left complex bundle of tissues that aid with electrical impulses, ending with the Purkinje fibers, which are highly conductive myofibers.

Innervations of the cardiac cells commence in the SA node, which is located in the right atrium. Both the atria contract in response to the SA node. The ventricles contract next in response to innervations from the AV node. The electrical impulse travels down the complex bundles and into the Bundle of His. Electricity then flows through the right and left conduction myofibers (Purkinje fibers). In a normal healthy heart, the SA node fires at a rate of about 60–100 beats per minute. If the SA node is unable to pace the heart appropriately, the AV node takes over at a more reduced speed. The heart is able to pace itself even at the lowest levels (the Purkinje fibers) but at a rate of about 30 beats per minute.

This entire cycle is captured in a wave form. When the ventricles relax, at the end of their innervations, repolarization occurs and this is evidenced by the T wave. As the action potential picks up again, the SA node (depolarization) and the AV node fire electrical responses that are seen via the P wave, the QRS complex ending with repolarization, the T wave.

Myocardial Infarction (MI)

The risk factors for MI include coronary artery disease (CAD) and local insufficiency of oxygen flow to the myocardium. The insufficiency may be due to loss of circulating blood volume which carries nutrients and oxygen to the myocardium and may set the stage for tissue necrosis. Oftentimes, the necrosis causes irreversible damage to cardiac cells that despite early interventions, cannot be salvaged. The myocytes within the subendocardium potentiate a wave-like pattern of cell death that extends throughout. Because of the extent of damage, it often takes 20 to 40 minutes for tissue death to occur and up to 6 hours post tissue death for the myocardial infarction (MI) to complete itself. Coronary arterial disease is the major cause of MIs.

The death of the cardiac muscle: when myocardium cells die, infarctions occur and can often extend to other areas of the cardiac muscle. Because it is the single most common cause of death in the United States, current and up-to-date knowledge regarding assessment, intervention, and prevention are important.

Loss of myocardium tissue affects the heart muscle in other ways. There is reduced wall motion, the atrium and most specifically the ventricles lose their compliancy and potentiate the possibility for left ventricular hypertrophy because of the excess demands. In addition, there is moderate stroke volume reduction with a reduced ejection fracture, which places patients already at risk (congestive heart failure, incompetent valves).

Although myocardial infarcts can affect many of the coronary arteries, the ones most affected are the left anterior descending artery, the right coronary artery, and the left circumflex which surrounds the cardiac muscle. Infarcts along these arteries not only cause tissue necrosis but they also cause damage to their surrounding areas, known as ischemia. These two factors, necrosis and ischemia, determine the overall amount of area injury.

Coronary arterial disease is certainly a contributory factor in MIs because of plaque buildup, but there are times when nonatherosclerotic changes cause MIs. They include congenital malformations of the vascular system, the release of emboli within the body (heart, lungs, or brain), weakening of the vessel walls (the aorta), chronic arterial inflammation (diabetes mellitus [DM], smoking), vessel spasms, use of illicit drugs such as cocaine, hypercoagulopathies (polycythemia vera or V Leiden [Factor 5]) deficiency (Table 3–1).

TABLE 3–1 ESC/ACC Definition of Myocardial Infarction

Criteria for acute MI

1. Typical rise and gradual fall (troponin) or more rapid rise and fall (CK-MB) of biochemical markers of myocardial necrosis with at least one of the following:

   a. Ischemic symptoms

   b. Development of pathologic Q waves on the ECG

   c. ECG changes indicative of ischemia (ST segment elevation or depression)

   d. Coronary artery intervention (e.g., coronary angioplasty)

2. Pathologic findings of an AMI

Criteria for established MI

Any one of the following criteria satisfies the diagnosis for established MI:

1. Development of new pathologic Q waves on serial ECGs. The patient may or may not remember previous symptoms. Biochemical markers of myocardial necrosis may have normalized, depending on the length of time that has passed since the infarct developed.

2. Pathologic findings of a healed or healing MI

MI, myocardial infarction; CK-MB, myocardial muscle kinase isoenzyme; ECG, electrocardiogram.
Adapted from Beller GA, et al. *J Am Coll Cardiol*. 2000;36:957. Copyright Elsevier 2000.

Clinical Manifestations

Symptoms of MI are evident once tissue ischemia has occurred. The patient may or may not exhibit the symptoms detailed below. Keep in mind that women and men present MI symptomatology differently from each other. Symptoms include the following:

- Pain in the chest described as burning, a tight band around the chest, crushing, or squeezing in nature. The pain is not relieved by conventional methods. It is persistent and lasts greater than 30 minutes.

- There may or may not be radiation of the pain from the chest to other areas of the body. If it radiates, the arms, middle of the back, neck, jaw, and shoulder may also be painful.

- Consider the elderly in whom because of neuropathy, the chest pain of an MI may not be present.

- Feelings of impending doom, anxiety, fear, confusion, or agitation may be present

- Shortness of breath, dyspnea, fatigue, and restlessness due to reduced oxygenation

- In women, the MI symptomatology may also include abdominal discomfort, fatigue, heartburn, or back pain, with fatigue being the greatest indicator.
- Nausea, vomiting
- Pallor, diaphoresis
- Changes in the level of consciousness (LOC) without other causes
- Syncope or near syncope episodes

Diagnostic Tests

Diagnostic tests are geared to determine the level of tissue ischemia, the presence of valvular disorders, and more specifically left ventricle assessment, which may be contributing to the lack of oxygen and the presence of arrhythmias. Blood work is also part of the expected workup specifically to assess for cardiac tissue breakdown. The tests include:

- Blood work: elevations in creatine kinase, lipids, creatine kinase–MB (CK-MB, which are specific to cardiac tissue), troponin I, troponin T, myoglobinuria (all the elevations result from the destruction of cardiac tissue and its associated release of proteins and enzymes into the bloodstream), increased white blood cell counts (inflammatory response), arterial blood gases (ABGs)
- Possible coronary interventions: percutaneous transluminal coronary angioplasty (PTCA), angioplasty, stents, atherectomy, left ventricular assist devices, or cardiac bypass
- Diagnostic testing include: electrocardiographic (ECG) tracings, echocardiogram

Complications

Complications of MI are catastrophic and are best prevented or minimized by strict cardiac monitoring and continuous assessment of the patient. They include the following:

- Abnormal rhythms are a common complication of MIs. These dysrhythmias account for almost 90% of all conduction disturbances post-MIs. Common dysrhythmias include ventricular tachycardia, premature ventricular contractions, ventricular fibrillation, atrial fibrillation/atrial flutter, right/left bundle branch blocks, first- and second-degree heart blocks, complete heart blocks, or sinus bradycardia/tachycardia.

- Rupture of ventricle wall is another complication with serious effects. The left ventricle under a great deal of pressure ruptures, potentiating cardiac tamponade. The heart is unable to fill with blood appropriately, and a precipitous drop in blood pressure occurs. The patient exhibits cardiogenic shock with progressive and worsening heart failure.

- Thromboembolisms occur as fragments of necrotic tissue float out of the cardiac muscle flowing to the brain, kidneys, spleen, or the mesenteric arterial system. Although venous embolisms are not a direct cause of MIs, they do occur as lethargy and fatigue from congestive heart failure patients encourages altered mobility, deep vein thrombosis, and pulmonary emboli.

- Aneurysm of the ventricles, which is an out-pouching or ballooning of the ventricle due to muscle weakness and fatigue, fills up with blood, clots, and other debris excreted by the necrotic cardiac tissue. At times, this debris may venture out into the systemic circulation, potentiating thromboembolisms. At other times, the aneurysm causes the ventricle to rupture, causing cardiac tamponade and death of the patient.

Nursing Interventions

Acute Phase:

- If patient is complaining of chest pain, expect that an immediate ECG will be ordered
- Start an intravenous line if not already in place
- Sit the patient upright, preferably at a 45-degree angle
- Assess respiratory status
- Take a set of vital signs; record and monitor vitals
- Get an oxygenation saturation rate and start low-flow oxygen if <92% (2 L/minute), record and monitor continuously
- Assess level of pain and medicate accordingly. Morphine is often the drug of choice. Keep Narcan readily available as morphine's major side effect is respiratory depression.
- Maintain bedrest and NPO (nothing by mouth) status
- Provide emotional support and do not leave patient alone
- Call for supportive help if patient is not stabilized

Postacute Phase:

- Teach patient signs and symptoms of MI

- Review discharge instructions—primary care/cardiologist follow-up appointments, dietitian/nutritionist consult, medications (use, timing, importance, side effects), activity tolerance levels and slowly increasing activity over time, possible cardiac rehabilitation transfer if patient deconditioned because of the coronary event.

- Need for continuous blood work assessment if on anticoagulants: Coumadin and electrolytes monitoring: potassium, sodium, calcium, and magnesium

Hypertension

Known as the "silent killer" disease, hypertension affects many Americans. Factors such as lifestyle, hereditary, comorbidities, sleep deprivation, high sodium intake in diets, and atherosclerotic disease are significant contributors to the development of increased pressures.

As the left ventricle contracts and forces blood up and into the aorta, which then distributes the oxygenated blood throughout the human body, arterial pressures are exerted for this to occur effectively. The pressures rise and fall in response to the baroreceptors that make note of the filling and emptying chambers of the heart. The systolic pressure, which should measure at or below 120 mm Hg, and the diastolic pressure, which should measure at or below 80 mm Hg, correspond to an even balance of force and exertion on the vessel walls. The differences between the systolic and diastolic pressures equate the pulse pressures, which are indicators of arterial blood flow. In addition, what determines the end values of pressure is the cardiac workload cycle, also known as the cardiac output (CO). Cardiac output is expressed as BP (blood pressure) = CO × SV (stroke volume, i.e., the amount of blood that is forced out of the ventricle and through the aorta upon every beat of the heart). Peripheral vascular resistance works with cardiac output and stroke volume as a force of resistance from the arterial walls in response to blood volume. Hence, blood pressure is regulated or maintained by a combination of cardiac output, stroke volume, and vascular resistance.

Two types of primary hypertension exist. The first is essential hypertension, whose etiology is unknown. However, there is increasing knowledge that associated factors are contributory to essential hypertension. They include heredity, obesity, sleep apnea, advancing age, ethnicity/race, renal changes, neural mechanisms, and increased sodium intake. Other possible contributory factors include diabetes mellitus, type A personalities, smoking, and lack of physical exercise.

Secondary hypertension has etiologic causes centering primarily on renal disorders, renovascular irregularities, acute/chronic glomerulonephritis, stenosis of the renal arteries, or atherosclerosis. Others include adrenal disorders such as Cushing disease or pheochromocytomas, pregnancy, use of oral contraceptives, chronic alcohol abuse, or coarctation of the aorta.

Malignant hypertension is a rapidly increasing hypertensive episode that is difficult to control. Because of its rapid onset, oftentimes, irreversible end organ damage to the brain, eyes, heart, and kidneys occur. In the brain, cerebrovascular accidents occur; in the eyes, retinal hemorrhages; in the heart, congestive heart failure; and in the kidney, possible acute/chronic renal failure.

Clinical Manifestations

Elevated venous and arterial pressures cause consistent and persistent damage to the vasculature of the human body systems. Signs and symptoms vary in degree of presentation and, at times, the symptomatology of hypertension is silent—hence the "silent killer syndrome." When symptoms are present, they include the following:

- Early morning headaches
- Dull aching headaches throughout the day
- Visual disturbances
- Orthostatic hyper- or hypotensive change
- Fatigue
- Proteinuria

Diagnostic Tests

There are no specific diagnostic tests to exclude or diagnose hypertension except for the direct measurement of blood pressure. However, additional supportive tests are used to evaluate the end organ damage hypertension causes. These tests include the following:

- Laboratory tests: comprehensive panel, lipids, hepatic levels, erythrocyte sedimentation rate (ESR), C-reactive protein
- Radiographic studies: magnetic resonance imaging (MRI), computed tomography (CT), x-ray, and ultrasonography (brain, kidney, heart)
- Ophthalmoscopic examination for hypertensive retinopathy

Nursing Interventions

- Assess patient's baseline blood pressure. Two to three readings in a quiet and calm environment will give the nurse a good estimation of blood pressure values.

- Recognize which patient may exhibit "white coat syndrome," which is a paradoxical elevation in blood pressure due to the presence of a health care professional. In this case, ask the patient to log his or her blood pressure in the patient's own time and bring the log for evaluation.

- Determine what risk factors are present in the patient. Consider race/ethnicity, diet, weight, comorbidities, exercise levels, levels of stress, other medications, and psychological status.

- Teach patient important lifestyle modifications that will help reduce blood pressure effectively: low-sodium diet, increasing exercise, awareness and determination to care for self, holistic medication support such as garlic, reducing weight, and managing levels of stress by increasing activities that relax the mind and body.

- Teach patients to take their prescribed medications and awareness that although blood pressure levels will be more manageable with blood pressure medications, stopping the medications will revert to increased pressure again.

- Teach patients the importance of monitoring side effects of hypertensive medications: hypotension. They should not fail to report dizziness, syncope, or falls to their health care provider. Remind the patient to shift positions slowly to avoid orthostatic changes.

- Teach patients the importance of follow-up appointments with cardiology, ophthalmology, endocrinology (if DM present), and nephrology (if renal impairment noted).

- If hospitalized, monitor therapeutic drug effects, maintain adequate intake and outputs (I&Os), and weigh the patient daily.

- Encourage smoking cessation programs and actively help patient set goals to stop smoking.

Complications

Hypertension carries significant complications commonly known as complications of end organ damage. The organs include kidney, heart, eyes, and brain. Sequelae of damages to these organs is compounded as eventually other body systems become indirectly damaged because of hypertension.

- Kidney: reduced renal arterial blood flow and chronic inflammation of the renal vessels due to increased pressures and loss of flexibility along with decreased blood flow place the kidney at risk to fail. Kidney failure commences as renal insufficiency progresses into acute or chronic renal failure over time. Nephrosclerosis develops from chronic hypertension. African Americans are most at risk because of other complicating comorbidities, including diabetes mellitus (diabetic nephropathy).

- Heart: the development of atherosclerosis over time predisposes sensitive cardiac vessels to dysfunction. In addition, sensitive cardiac tissue suffers. Over time, congestive heart failure develops, incidence of stroke increases, and the development of peripheral arterial and venous disease takes it course. Keep in mind, like the renal system, comorbidities such as smoking, EtOH (ethyl alcohol) abuse, obesity, sedentary lifestyle, and diet (high-fat/cholesterol) play a significant role too. Cardiomyopathy is another complication of uncontrolled hypertension. Over time, the cardiac muscle has to work harder against systemic elevated pressures and, because it is a muscle after all, it will increase in size. The left ventricle is the muscle mostly affected. Sudden death, congestive heart failure, valvular dysfunction, and cardiac dysrhythmias occur.

- Brain: increasing pressures predispose the patient to have elevated pressures within a tightly closed cranium that at times cannot handle the extra load. Cerebral hemorrhages or ischemic events thus occur. Although elevated pressures systemically impair brain function, concurrently, atherosclerotic changes to the small vessels in the brain contribute to hypoperfusion, which contributes to irreversible changes within the white matter of the brain.

- Eyes: hypertensive retinopathy places the patient at risk for visual acuity changes, changes in intraocular pressures, and subsequent vision loss due to reduced arterial and venous perfusion. The microvascular system behind the retina succumbs to reduced perfusion, becoming sclerotic and thickening or buckling the eye globe.

Angina Pectoris

Pain, pain, and more pain. Angina pectoris is a broad descriptive definition for various types of pain experienced by patients. The different types of anginal pain include stable angina, variant or Prinzmetal angina, silent ischemic, and unstable angina.

Supply-and-demand balances between availability of oxygen and circulation contribute to the cardiac pain known as angina. When a patient senses anginal pain it is because of reduced oxygen availability to the cardiac tissue that is increasingly demanding more oxygen. At the cellular level, the cardiac cells require oxygen in order to transport necessary cellular respiration to all body systems. Simply put, any condition that changes the integrity of the lumen of any vessel will cause that vessel to deliver less and less blood to an organ. Atherosclerotic changes because of plaque formation are important contributory factors.

The human body is remarkable in that it can autoregulate itself to assist in the maintenance of homeostasis. It can do so for long periods of time. In this case, autoregulation of coronary blood flow through the relaxation and constriction of blood keeps the blood flowing smoothly to all necessary organs. However, homeostasis over time in a body that is stressed causes an imbalance. The powerful vasodilator adenosine is responsible along with other important agents and baroreceptor mechanisms in regulating resistance. When adenosine can no longer maintain the ebb and flow of blood in order to meet the metabolic demands of the body, ischemia develops. Once ischemia continues, diminished blood flow dominates and it is manifested in the patient as angina. Keep in mind that ischemic changes are reversible and cardiac cells can be repaired if blood flow is returned to the area immediately.

Although the heart itself, if manipulated, does not cause pain, the pain felt in angina due to ischemic changes is probably due to the release of lactic acid from damaging cardiac muscles. Lactic acid acts as an irritant to the nerve endings sending messages through the sympathetic nervous system. The accompanying pains felt in cardiac ischemia, though not labeled angina in and of itself, is due to sympathetic nerve irritation along the thoracic and cervical ganglia up and down the spinal cord. This is the reason that patients with MI feel referred pain in addition to anginal pain along the left arm, jaw, stomach, esophagus, and middle of the back.

Clinical Manifestations

Pain is the presenting symptom. Below is a brief discussion of the different types of anginal pain and their particular characteristics:

- Stable angina: patient will tell you his or her pain is predictable. The pain usually occurs after sexual activity, ingestion of a heavy meal, and increasing activity levels. Hallmark is that once the behavior is discontinued, the pain subsides.

- Variant/Prinzmetal: patient will tell you the pain is exacerbated during the night hours, oftentimes waking him or her up from deep sleep possibly because of vasospasm.

- Silent ischemic: absence of chest pain with noted cardiac dysrhythmias usually discovered during exercise stress tests, in the patient with advancing age or in the diabetic patient due to increasing neuropathy

- Unstable angina: oftentimes seen in patients whose anginal pain has progressed from stable angina to unstable angina. The patient will alert the nurse that the pain is getting worse over time, with increasing severity and frequency. If left untreated, unstable angina will lead to ischemia and eventual infarction.

Diagnostic Tests

Perhaps the most important test for angina is ECG tracings in combination with other diagnostic data acquired throughout the cardiac events. Close monitoring and evaluation of diagnostic tests by competent health care providers improve outcomes and decrease incidence of complications of angina.

- Serum: CK, CK-MBs, lactate dehydrogenase (LD), LD isoenzymes, myoglobin, aspartate transaminase (AST)/alanine transaminase (ALT), troponins (I and T), calcium, phosphate, blood urea nitrogen/creatinine ratio (BUN:Cr), lipids (low-density lipoprotein [LDL], high-density lipoprotein [HDL], total cholesterol), HbA1c, thyroid

- Stress tests: treadmill exercise, dobutamine/adenosine, stress echocardiogram, nuclear stress test

- Angiography of the coronary arteries

- Holter monitoring as an outpatient

Nursing Interventions

- Vital sign assessment

- With angina as with any other type of pain, a full comprehensive assessment of the pain is warranted: length of time, location of pain, frequency, what precipitates it, what makes it better, what was the patient doing when pain presented, qualify/quantify the pain

- Hemodynamic cardiac assessment: ECG tracings, cardiovascular status, labs, intake/output, oxygen therapy

- Administration of appropriate medications
- Reduction of psychosocial presentations that affect cardiac status: stress, anxiety, depression, fear, role dependency, inability to meet family/personal needs, body image disturbance
- Proper patient position to maximize lung capacity with frequent repositioning to minimize secretion stasis
- Patient and family teaching: signs/symptoms of cardiac complications associated with angina pain, importance with medication compliancy, follow-up appointments as needed, balance of activity and exercise, and avoiding precipitating factors that produce anginal pain
- Need to reach out for help (911) when symptoms are not readily manageable with treatment plans initiated by health care provider

Complications

With angina, targeted complications include signs and symptoms of congestive heart failure, irregular heart rhythms, and myocardial ischemia/infarction.

- Congestive heart failure (CHF): management and assessment of the important signs and symptoms of CHF are required. Assessing lung sounds, vascular sounds, edema (pulmonary, peripheral and ascites), oxygen saturation (SaO_2), vital signs should be continuous and assertive management and intervention of hypertensive presentations should be included.
- Arrhythmias: Instability of the cardiac muscle causes irritability and pain (angina). Cardiac monitoring should be consistent and transfer of the patient to a dedicated monitoring unit (telemetry) may be required. Arrhythmias can range from benign (infrequent premature ventricular contractions [PVCs]) to tachy/bradyarrhythmias that cause hemodynamic instability.
- Myocardial ischemia/infarction: cardiac damage or eventual cardiac tissue death due to reduction in blood flow because of obstruction causes the angina pain felt by patients. The ischemia/infarction destroys once-viable tissue and when the healing process commences, nonpliant scar tissue develops, further compromising cardiac output and leading to angina pain and other complications associated with myocardial damage.

Atherosclerosis

A large amount of sludge clotting up the arterial walls is the basic tenet for atherosclerosis. Fibrofatty plaque is the main culprit for this disease presentation. Many factors increase the incidence of this process and will be discussed next. Particular sites commonly found to accumulate fibrofatty plaques include the internal carotid arteries, the proximal coronary arteries, the abdominal aorta and iliac arteries, the thoracic aorta, femoral and popliteal arteries, and finally the vertebral, basilar, and middle cerebral arteries.

The development of atherosclerosis is a multistep process. It commences with endothelial cell injury along the arterial wall (because of a host of complicating factors: increasing age, being male, familial disposition to lipid metabolism, a family history of coronary arterial disease, smoking, obesity, diabetes (diabesity), chronic uncontrolled hypertension, low levels of HDL with high levels of LDLs, and chronic inflammatory diseases). This process is followed by the cascade of inflammatory agents (macrophages, lymphocytes, platelets, leukocytes, monocytes and cellular debris and lipoproteins). An accumulation of these debris forms lesions, and the foundation for plaque structures to form is solidified.

Lipid-laden materials form lesions that obscure arterial walls. There are three basic forms of these lipid-laden plaques: those that are consistent with fatty streaks (present at birth and become stable around the mid-20s), fibrous atheromatous plaques, and complicated lesions, which are a combination of both these plaques. Made of intra- and extracellular lipids, the lesions that cause the most destruction are the fibrous atheromatous lesions. The growth and proliferation of these plaques which are gray to translucent in color cause a thickening within the intima lumen of the arterial wall. This in turn sets off a cascade of inflammatory responses (presence of macrophages, lymphocytes, and necrotic smooth muscle cell debris) that assists in arterial stenosis, encroachment of the arterial wall, and eventual occlusion of the artery. Surrounding the outer wall of the fibrous lesion is a fibrous cap that appears smooth and intact. In females, because of the smoothness of this fibrous cap, occluding lesions may not be readily detected. The development of thrombosis is inevitable as the presence of fibrous plaque formation and its sequelae are allowed to proliferate. Turbulent blood flow complicates the disease process. In and around the fibrous lesion, focal lesions may also be detected.

Clinical Manifestations

The resulting clinical manifestations of atherosclerotic vessels are dependent on the location of the occlusion and the extent of the occlusion. Clinical manifestations are fluid in that each correlate with the degree of vessel damage. Vessels that are smaller manifest symptoms earlier than larger vessels. Small vessels hemorrhage, rupture, or develop aneurysms. Larger vessels such as the aorta weaken over time, developing aneurysms as well. Medium-size vessels such as the cerebral arteries cause distal ischemia and infarction. Because of the vascularity within the heart, brain, kidneys, lower extremities, and mesenteric areas, these organs will demonstrate damage quickly.

- Vessel narrowing
- Vessel obstruction
- Thrombosis and emboli formation
- Vessel endothelium damage

Diagnostic Tests

- Coronary arteriography: detects and determines plaque formation and extent of occlusion
- ECG tracings for important changes to an ischemic heart: ST depression or abnormal T waves, such as T-wave inversion
- Serum: CK, CK-MBs, LD, LD isoenzymes, myoglobin, AST/ALT, troponins (I and T), calcium, phosphate, BUN:Cr, and lipids (LDL, HDL, total cholesterol)
- Stress tests: treadmill exercise, dobutamine/adenosine, stress echocardiogram, and nuclear stress test

Nursing Interventions

- Vital signs assessment is important to monitor for changes in blood pressure that can occur with the presence of plaque buildup
- Administration of medications: statins, niacin, aspirin, anticoagulants
- Administer oxygen to prevent hypoxia
- Hemodynamic monitoring for unstable presentation of disease: chest pain, decreasing oxygen availability, increase/decrease in blood pressure, cyanosis, feelings of impending doom, and signs/symptoms of stroke

- Reduction of psychosocial presentations that affect cardiac status: stress, anxiety, depression, fear, role dependency, inability to meet family/personal needs, body image disturbance

Complications

- Stroke: hemorrhagic or embolic due to release/rupture of affected arteries
- Myocardial infarction: cardiac damage or eventual cardiac tissue death due to reduction in blood flow. The ischemia/infarction destroys once-viable tissue and when the healing process commences, nonpliant scar tissue develops, further compromising cardiac output, leading to angina pain and other complications associated with myocardial damage.
- Angina pain

Congestive Heart Failure

The heart is a myogenic muscular organ (an organ that can contract) that is capable of providing adequate circulation to all organs of the human body. It has a mass of approximately 250–350 g and is about the size of an adult fist. Around the heart is a protective sac called the pericardium. It serves to protect and cushion the heart from trauma and it helps keep the heart anchored into place beneath the sternal wall. Three main layers comprise the heart: the epicardium (outer layer), the myocardium (middle layer), and the innermost level, the endocardium. The four corresponding valves of the heart—the aortic valve, the pulmonic valve, the mitral valve, and the tricuspid valve—pulsate with rhythmic precision opening and closing as blood is shunted from the body to the heart, the lungs, and then back out to systemic circulation.

In congestive heart failure, the normal pathophysiology of the heart is disrupted. In and of itself, it is not a disease process but more a presentation of signs and symptoms either systemically or in the pulmonary vasculature that demonstrates the heart's inability to pump enough blood into, through, and then out of the heart.

Right-sided and left-sided are the two types of cardiogenic failures of the heart. There are various causes for heart failure. Intrinsically, heart failure can occur because of MIs, cardiomyopathy (long-standing hypertension), congenital heart disease, valvular disorders, and tamponade (cardiac/pericarditis). Extrinsic causes of heart failure include systemic hypertension, chronic obstructive pulmonary disease, pulmonary embolism, anemia, thyrotoxicosis, metabolic/respiratory acid-base disorders, dysrhythmias, drug toxicities, and metabolic diseases.

In diagnosing and managing heart failure, it is important to understand the four classifications of heart failure.

Class I	No symptoms noted with normal daily activity
Class II	Symptoms noted with normal daily activities but they subside with rest
Class III	Symptoms noted with minimal activity; may or may not be symptom-free at rest
Class IV	Symptoms usually present at rest and are worsened by any type of activity

(Courtesy: New York Heart Association Functional Classification of Heart Failure)

Heart failure or congestive heart failure (CHF) can occur over a long period of time or it can occur as an acute process. Overload and the inability of the heart to sustain that overload due to weakness contribute to the failure. In continued stressful cardiac situations, the heart's myogenic capability lessens, thereby reducing cardiac output. Predictable responses to the loss of cardiac output includes release of renin from the juxtaglomerular cells (to help blood pressure rise), increased reflex sympathetic activity (to help jump-start the muscle), and an increased drawing out of oxygen from peripheral cells in response to declining O_2 levels. Because of this increase, the heart, like any other muscle, increases in size and volume. Hypertrophy or cardiomegaly occurs. Heart rate is often elevated as the heart has to pump against more resistance and more volume. Both failures present with backward and forward effects of the circulatory compromise they cause. All are discussed below (Figure 3–1).

Left-Sided Failure

Left-sided failure results from overloading of volume within the left ventricle, and sometimes this can also cause overfilling of the left atria. Because the ejection fraction of an overloaded left ventricle is ineffective, the pulmonary veins and the pulmonary capillary bed become congested with blood. At some point, the pressure of the blood causes a "backward effect" and the blood passes across the pulmonary vascular and into the alveoli. When the lymphatic drainage system can no longer handle the movement of the excess fluid from the lungs into the lymphatic circulation, acute pulmonary edema

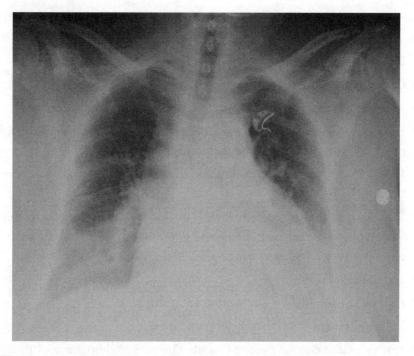

FIGURE 3–1 • Cardiomegaly with pulmonary venous congestion and bilateral pleural effusions. (Reproduced with permission from Usatine RP, et al. *The Color Atlas of Family Medicine*. New York: McGraw-Hill; 2009, figure 46-1. Courtesy of Kansas University Medical Center.)

occurs. Pulmonary edema can occur over time or it can be an acute process known as flash pulmonary edema. Gas exchange is severely impaired. Respiratory support and prompt interventions are required in order to prevent respiratory arrest/failure. The forward effects of left ventricular failure occur when the left ventricle fails to push out sufficient blood through the aorta. Perfusion to tissues of the body decreases. Baroreceptors along many important blood vessels including the aorta signal that insufficient blood is available; thus, systemic blood pressure decreases. Vasoconstriction ensues from the stimulated renin-angiotensin-aldosterone loop. Water and sodium are held on to tightly by the body. Extracellular fluid volume begins to increase and, subsequently, there is an increase in the total blood volume along with an increase in systemic blood pressure.

Clinical Manifestations (Left-Sided Failure)

The clinical manifestations vary because of either the chronicity of the disease or the acute nature of the disease. In chronic disease, the body has become more adaptable to the changes in blood volume and respiratory demand.

- Dyspnea is an early indicator of left-sided failure
- Oxygenation saturation begins to decline
- Respiratory rates increase in response to the drop in oxygenation
- Fatigue, weakness (both due to the extra work of breathing/breathlessness), and dizziness (due to hypoxia to the brain)
- Disorientation, confusion, and changes to the level of consciousness can occur
- Because of the increased levels of aldosterone (renin-angiotensin-aldosterone mechanism), K^+ loss is potentiated; therefore, patients will exhibit muscle weakness and possible dysrhythmias
- Orthopnea is pronounced
- Extra heart sounds are auscultated (S^3 gallop)
- Pulsus alternans develops
- Paroxysmal nocturnal dyspnea (acute episodes of dyspnea nocturnally)
- And in the case of acute/flash pulmonary edema: coughing, pink frothy/bloody sputum, marked shortness of breath, rales, exaggerated breathing patterns, increased venous pressure, anxiety, rapid weak pulse, decreased urinary output, and ashen or cyanotic skin that is cool to touch

Right-Sided Failure

The left side of the heart is the main denominator of right-sided failure. The right heart fails simply because of the increased pulmonary pressure exerted by increased fluid accumulations. The backward effects of right-sided failure occur as there is a decrease in the emptying of the right ventricle. As this happens, there is increased volume and end-diastolic pressures within the right ventricle. The right atrium pressures also elevate. There is increased volume and pressure within the great veins. This tends to increase the systemic venous circulation, overloading the tissues and vasculature at the other end. Hepatomegaly, splenomegaly, ascites, peripheral edema, and distended neck veins are all the end results of the increased pressures and the backing up of fluid. The forward effects of right-sided failure occur as the volume from the right ventricle decreases, and there is a decreased return to the left atrium with subsequent decreased cardiac output. All of the forward effects of left-sided heart failure are produced with the ultimate effect of increased blood volume and vasoconstriction.

Clinical Manifestations (Right-Sided Failure)

Unlike left-sided failure, the clinical manifestations are more systemic than pulmonary although there are eventual pulmonary sequelae for right-sided failure.

- Dependent, pitting edema (peripheral)
- Hepatosplenomegaly
- Jaundice
- Coagulation problems
- Ascites
- Jugular vein distention
- When pulmonary system is affected—shortness of breath, pleural effusions, dyspnea

Diagnostic Tests: Diagnostic Tests are Similar in Both Types of Failure

- Labs: blood chemistry and B-type natriuretic peptide (BNP). Keep in mind that BNP is a 32–amino acid polypeptide that is excreted by the heart's ventricles when excessive stress and pressure are exerted by the heart during failure. Consistent elevation of BNP is a diagnostic clue for failure and a poorer prognosis. Electrolytes must be monitored carefully, as digoxin is a drug of choice in failure. Keep in mind that high Ca^{2+} levels, low Mg^{2+} levels, and hypokalemia can alter digoxin's therapeutic effects.
- Urinalysis: myoglobinuria, proteinuria, hematuria, cast debris
- Chest x-ray, echocardiogram, ECG
- Hemodynamic monitoring: pulmonary artery wage pressure (PAWP), central venous pressure (CVP), pulmonary artery pressure (PAP)
- Arterial blood gases

Nursing Interventions: Interventions are Based on Priority ABCs

- Assess cardiopulmonary status consistently and frequently
- Monitor vital signs remembering that small changes make a difference in the cardiopulmonary status of this patient
- Oxygen therapy as needed and titrated to oxygen saturation levels
- Venous access important: intravenous fluids, emergency medications
- Positioning is important for better lung expansion and to decrease immobilization of pulmonary secretions that can compromise pulmonary function: semi-Fowler
- Hydration is important; however, fluid restriction may be required
- Pulmonary toileting is priority: suction, deep breathing, repositioning every 1–2 hours, use of pillows for comfort and to decrease fatigue secondary to breathing
- Daily weights monitoring carefully for weight gain/loss of 2 lbs. or more
- Assess lower extremities, jugular veins, and abdomen for fluid retention
- Teach importance of follow-up: medications, follow-up appointments, daily weighing, fluid restriction if indicated, diet (low sodium, low cholesterol), teach patient signs and symptoms of fluid overload (increased difficulty breathing, edema in lower extremities, activity intolerance)
- Administer medications: digoxin, diuretics, nesiritide (Natrecor), which is a recombinant clone of BNP and is used to supplement the loss of BNP during cardiac damage secondary to failure.
- Indwelling urinary catheter to assist in monitoring fluid output

Complications

Left-sided failure: Acute pulmonary edema that is life threatening and death can occur within minutes of the pulmonary edema especially if the fluid backup is sudden and severe. Marked shortness of breath, anxiety, and changes in the vital signs occur in succession. If not managed effectively, respiratory failure/arrest may occur. Monitor patient carefully for cardiogenic shock. Patients with heart failure are usually started on digoxin (Lanoxin), a cardiac glycoside that increases/strengthens cardiac contractions in the presence of failure. Digoxin carries a tight therapeutic range, so toxicity can occur. Monitor for signs and symptoms: yellow vision, heart block, tachycardia/bradycardia, and/or abdominal pain.

Right-sided failure: Massive peripheral edema secondary to engorgement of the venous and portal systems may lead to organ failure/compromise. Eventual respiratory failure/arrest is possible. Monitor for digoxin toxicity.

Rheumatic Fever

Affecting a younger population set (ages 5 through 15), rheumatic fever may occur after an inflammatory insult to the body. Infections of the throat with group A β-hemolytic streptococci (gram-positive *Streptococcus pyogenes*) left untreated may be the culprit.

Although the complete etiology of rheumatic fever is unknown, it is thought that its appearance is an immunologic response to the infection. Because of the introduction of the gram-positive bacteria, streptococcal antigenic responses may activate cytotoxic T cells that may cross-react with cardiac cells, causing a possible acute inflammatory response of the heart. Rheumatic fever can also affect other body systems: musculoskeletal system, the integumentary system, and the nervous system. Chronic bouts of rheumatic fever may lead to valvular disease. There is suspicion that there might be an increased genetic disposition to the development of rheumatic fever.

The musculoskeletal association of rheumatic fever occurs because of excessive accumulation of exudative synovial fluid causing synovitis with associated subcutaneous nodules along the joint tracks. Cardiac presentation is more of a pancarditis where the endocardium, the myocardium, and the pericardium are affected. When viewed microscopically, Aschoff-Geipel bodies or nodules are present within the heart. The presences of these lesions are consistent with rheumatic fever. Vegetative changes known as verrucae are noted along the leaflets of the cardiac valves. All four valves are susceptible to the vegetative changes as well as the chordae tendineae causing edema, acute inflammation, and dysfunction. Over time, interadherence, scarring, and shortening of these structures will occur. Sydenham chorea (St. Vitus dance) presentation indicates nervous system involvement of rheumatic fever. Gait disturbance, cognitive changes, and loss of fine/gross motor skills are common.

Clinical Manifestations

- Chronic/acute inflammatory arthritis in multiple joints that is migratory, meaning the inflammation shifts from joint to joint, dysarthria
- Development of nodules over the joints most especially of the hands, wrist, elbows
- Changes in vital signs: fever, tachycardia
- Rash along the torso and lower extremities that appear in concentric circles (erythema marginatum)
- Murmurs
- Abnormal gait, cognitive changes, loss of fine/gross motor skills

Diagnostic Tests

- Jones Criteria for Acute Rheumatic Fever: www.medicalcritera.com— two major criteria or one major and two minor criteria must be present in addition to the diagnosis of a streptococcal infection. *Major criteria*: carditis, polyarthritis, chorea, rash (erythema marginatum) or the presence of nodules over the joints. *Minor criteria*: fever (low or high grade), history of rheumatic fever, blood chemistries (elevated ESR and C-reactive proteins plus leukocyte presence), and ECG changes demonstrated dysfunctional atria (prolonged P-R intervals)
- Echocardiogram
- Throat culture (however, empiric commencement of antibiotics may be indicated)

Nursing Interventions

- Assess cardiopulmonary status, especially pulmonary status
- Monitor vital signs, intake and output
- Administer oxygen, intravenous fluids, antiinflammatory agents, antibiotics (penicillin, sulfadiazine, or erythromycin), keeping in mind that patients with chronic valvular disease may require prophylactic treatment with antibiotics for at least 5 years after the acute presentation.
- Pulmonary toileting: improve saturation and diminish risk of pneumonia

- Rest with periods of activity as tolerated to help reduce activity intolerance and encourage independence within limits
- Monitor for changes or disappearance of the presentations within the Jones Criteria
- Monitor for side effects, adverse effects, and therapeutic effects of the medications

Complications

- Development of rheumatic heart disease, which is permanent damage to the cardium because of chronicity of the inflammation.
- Stenosis and/or regurgitation of the valves.
- Damage to the heart muscle that may precipitate congestive heart failure, reduced cardiac output and pulmonary/systemic complications
- Dysrhythmias: atrial fibrillation, atrial flutter

Valvular Disorders

The heart functions through a series of processes that involve contraction of the heart muscle, coordinated movements of structures within the heart and electrical responses generated by shifts in electrolytes. Of the many structures within the heart, the four valves are the channels by which blood flows through and within the muscle to the lungs and to systemic circulation. Changes or alterations of the heart valves directly and indirectly affect cardiac output, causing a cascade of symptoms and other complications throughout the human body. The heart as mentioned has four valves: the aortic semilunar valve, the pulmonary semilunar valve, the tricuspid valve, and the bicuspid valve (also known as the mitral valve), which lie along the atrioventricular border.

There are two forms of disorders within the heart valves. The first is stenosis, which is the hardening and/or narrowing of the valve orifice. The stenotic valve decreases the amount of blood that flows between the chambers of the heart. Stenotic valves produce distention of the chambers of the heart. The second disorder is regurgitation, also known as the incompetent valve. The incompetent valve increases atrial and ventricle pressures because it does not effectively move all the blood from the chambers, causing stagnant blood to regurgitate or flow back into the left ventricle. This disorder also contributes to distention of the heart muscle and increases the work load of the heart.

As mentioned, the role of the valves is to direct the flow of blood. Stenotic or incompetent valves can develop through a mirage of disorders. Some include inflammation (such as rheumatic fever), congenital disorders, degenerative changes to the valves, or ischemic changes. Valvular disorders are least common among the pulmonary and tricuspid valves, probably because of the lower pressures of the right heart, and conversely the mitral and aortic valve will demonstrate more destructive changes because of the higher pressures of the left heart. The mitral valve and the aortic valve will be the two discussed here.

Mitral Valve Disorders

Stenosis

During the systolic/diastolic cycle, the stenotic mitral valve causes incomplete opening of the valve. The incomplete opening impairs the filling of the left ventricle and distention of the left atrium. Stenosis of the mitral valve is attributed to rheumatic fever. Over time, the stenosis progresses at an even pace, accelerating as the patient gets older. In understanding congestive heart failure, the stenotic mitral valve eventually dilates the left side of the heart, precipitating left-sided heart failure. When auscultating the mitral valve, a snap can be heard immediately after the S2 heart sound.

Clinical Manifestations: (Mitral Valve Stenosis)

- All symptoms of pulmonary congestion—orthopnea and nocturnal paroxysmal dyspnea
- Fatigue
- Chest pain
- Tachycardia
- Weakness
- Dysrhythmias: atrial irregularities (atrial fibrillation or atrial tachycardia). This predisposes the patient to thrombus formation and dislodgement (stroke).

Diagnostic Tests

- Angiography
- Chest x-ray

- Echocardiogram
- Cardiac catheterization

Nursing Interventions

- Cardiopulmonary assessment
- Oxygen therapy
- Monitoring vital signs
- Hemodynamic monitoring
- Labs: electrolytes, coagulation studies
- Arterial blood gases
- Medication administration: digoxin (Lanoxin), isosorbidedinitrate (Isordil), nitroglycerin, diuretic therapy; antiarrhythmics: amiodarone (Cordarone); anticoagulants (especially in the presence of atrial fibrillation): warfarin (Coumadin)
- Positioning: semi-Fowler
- Balance activity with rest

Complications

- Thrombosis development (stroke, transient ischemic attack [TIA])
- Right- and left-sided congestion heart failure
- Dysrhythmias: Atrial fibrillation
- Cardiac arrest

Regurgitation

The mitral valve cannot close completely; therefore blood trickles back into the left heart chamber. Persistent blood accumulation distends the chamber. Again, rheumatic fever may be a causative factor. Chordae tendineae dysfunction or stretching of the valve because the ventricle is dilated may also contribute to the regurgitating of the mitral valve. Heart pansystolic murmurs are common because of the left enlarged ventricle as well as a hyperdynamic left ventricle impulse.

Mitral valve prolapse is a common causative factor to the mitral valve regurgitation. Found more commonly in women than men, there is a suspected genetic disposition to its development. Patients with connective tissue disorders, osteogenesis imperfecta (soft, brittle bones), and Marfan syndrome have been suspected to develop. Changes within the mitral valve of mucinous degeneration cause the valve leaflets to become floppy and large, making them easy to prolapse or fall back into the left atrium during systole. The leaflets form a ballooning shape that billows within the chamber.

Clinical Manifestations: (Mitral Valve Regurgitation and Prolapse)

- Cardiomegaly, murmurs
- Fatigue
- Chest pain
- Weakness
- In mitral valve prolapse (possibly asymptomatic) but can also exhibit angina, dyspnea, fatigue, anxiety, tachycardia, and dizziness
- Dysrhythmias: atrial irregularities (atrial fibrillation or atrial tachycardia). This predisposes the patient to thrombus formation and dislodgement (stroke).
- Sudden death (although rare), especially if there is a family history

Diagnostic Tests

- Angiography
- Chest x-ray
- Echocardiogram
- Cardiac catheterization

Nursing Interventions

- Cardiopulmonary assessment
- Oxygen therapy
- Monitoring vital signs
- Hemodynamic monitoring
- Labs: electrolytes, coagulation studies
- Arterial blood gases
- Monitor pain levels consistently
- Assess for peripheral edema

- Administer: intravenous fluids
- Positioning: semi-Fowler
- Balance activity with rest
- Monitor for depression, anxiety, fear

Complications

- Pulmonary edema
- Right- and left-sided congestive heart failure
- Rupture of the fragile papillary muscles of the valve
- Embolism/thrombosis
- Dysrhythmias: atrial fibrillation

Aortic Valve Disorders

Stenosis

Because of the fibrotic valve, increased resistance to blood flow from the left ventricle into the massive aorta occurs. There are many factors that cause the valve orifice to stiffen. Congenital abnormalities make up the highest risk for the development of stenosis. However, over time, especially as patients are living longer, the normal wear and tear of years of opening and closing bring on calcifications that stiffen the valve. During the 8th and 9th decade of life, stenosis may present. Stenosis may become evident during the 6th and 9th decade of life if previous valvular disorders are present. Often more common in men than women, the changes seen within the aortic valve mimics changes of coronary arterial disease, especially in the presence of hyperlipidemia. Plaque buildup and chronic inflammation contribute to the stenotic process. Aortic stenosis develops over time, allowing the left heart to accommodate to the stiffening of the valve. Cardiomegaly is not uncommon. However, ejection fractions (EFs) are maintained because the left ventricle is still able to push out blood effectively.

Clinical Manifestations

- Chest pain
- Fainting (syncope or near syncope)

- Pulmonary congestion—orthopnea, paroxysmal nocturnal dyspnea
- Fatigue
- Weakness
- Murmurs

Diagnostic Tests

- Angiography
- Chest x-ray
- Echocardiogram
- Cardiac catheterization

Nursing Interventions

- Cardiopulmonary assessment
- Oxygen therapy
- Monitoring vital signs
- Hemodynamic monitoring
- Labs: electrolytes, coagulation studies
- Arterial blood gases
- Monitor pain levels consistently
- Assess for peripheral edema
- Administer: intravenous fluids
- Positioning: semi-Fowler
- Balance activity with rest
- Monitor for depression, anxiety, fear

Complications

- Left-sided congestive heart failure
- Pulmonary edema
- Cardiomegaly
- Dysrhythmias
- Infectious endocarditis

Regurgitation

Back flow of blood is the hallmark of regurgitation. With aortic incompetency, blood flows back into the left ventricle during the heart's resting period, diastole. Stroke volume is an expected response from the left ventricle because the left ventricle has to manage the leaking valve and the backflow of cleansed blood from the pulmonary arteries. Because of the increased pressures, backflow of blood into the pulmonary veins occurs, translating into pulmonary edema. Because of the blood flow dysfunction, systemic responses correlate to a reduced cardiac output. Heart rate increases and peripheral vascular resistance increases, all of which potentiate a worsening of the incompetency of the valve. Rheumatic fever, congenital abnormalities, connective tissue disorders, prolonged and unmanaged hypertension, trauma, or infectious endocarditis can also be causative factors.

Clinical Manifestations

- Sign and symptoms of left sided congestive heart failure
- Pulmonary congestion—orthopnea, dyspnea, paroxysmal nocturnal dyspnea
- Neck pain
- Chest pain—angina
- Tachycardia
- Murmurs

Diagnostic Tests

- Angiography
- Chest x-ray
- Echocardiogram
- Cardiac catheterization

Nursing Interventions

- Cardiopulmonary assessment
- Oxygen therapy
- Monitoring vital signs
- Hemodynamic monitoring
- Labs: electrolytes, coagulation studies

- Arterial blood gases
- Monitor pain levels consistently
- Assess for peripheral edema
- Administer: intravenous fluids
- Positioning: semi-Fowler
- Balance activity with rest
- Monitor for depression, anxiety, fear

Complications

- Heart failure
- Thrombosis/embolism (stroke, TIA)
- Cardiomegaly
- Infection

CASE STUDY: CARDIOVASCULAR

Hypertension: A Nurse Practitioner's Perspective

The nurse practitioner works at a local outpatient clinic. She has developed a professional rapport with her patients over the last few years and this rapport has solidified, offering a trusting relationship because she is of the same ethnicity as most of her patients and she speaks Spanish fluently.

One of the patients, who has been coming to the clinic for quite some time, has an appointment for today. The nurse practitioner notes that she cancelled her last two appointments, both of which were blood pressure checks. The nurse practitioner notes that two telephone attempts were documented reaching out to the patient regarding her missed appointments.

The medical assistant takes the patient into the room and takes her vitals. They are:

BP (blood pressure): 200/100 right, 180/100 left; HR (heat rate): 96; RR (respiration rate): 22; temperature: 98.6°F.

After a physical assessment by the nurse practitioner and follow-up blood pressure analysis, the following is documented:

BP: 190/100 right, 180/100 left; HR: 98; RR: 20; temperature: 98.6°F. Patient denies dizziness, syncope, chest pain, shortness of breath, dyspnea on exertion (DOE), or headache. However, on movement from chair to examination table, the patient becomes dizzy and almost falls to the ground. Reluctantly, she tells the nurse practitioner that she has, indeed, been more dizzy over the last few days and sometimes wakes up with a very painful headache. The nurse practitioner reviews the medications on the chart: lisinopril 10 mg QD (once daily), HCTZ (hydrochlorothiazide) 12.5 mg QD, simvastatin 20 mg QD, EC (enteric-coated) Aspirin 81 mg QD, and multivitamin QD. She asks the patient when was the last time she took her medications, most specifically, the blood pressure medicine.

The patient begins to laugh and the nurse practitioner is puzzled by the reaction. She states that the last time she took her BP medicines was 3 weeks ago. She claims that she took her blood pressure at a local pharmacy then and the reading was significantly lower than in the past, 148/90 mm Hg, although she cannot recall the exact reading. The patient says that the BP medicines were working and that the blood pressure had reduced; therefore, she would stop taking them because her friends told her too much medication is bad for the body.

QUESTIONS

Answer the following questions regarding the case study above:

1. What is the barrier to learning for this patient?
2. What should the nurse practitioner do next?
3. What should the nurse who supervises the appointments and subsequent blood pressure readings do next?
4. Is the blood pressure medication on target with appropriate blood pressure control or should it be changed? And if so, to what?
5. What are three important points to focus on in terms of patient education?
6. When should this patient be reevaluated by the nurse?
7. From the perspective of the nurse practitioner, are there any other important diagnostic tests that should be considered for this patient?

Suggested Readings

Battaglia M, Pewsner D, Jüni P, Egger M, Bucher HC, Bachmann LM. Accuracy of B-type natriuretic peptide tests to exclude congestive heart failure: systematic review of test accuracy studies. *Archives of Internal Medicine.* 2006;166:1073-1080.

Beth MN, Taylor J. Getting to the heart of aortic valvular disease. *Nursing.* 1998;28: 8-CC12.

Brown GE. Heart disease requiring surgical intervention: a continuum of nursing care. *Occup Health Nurs.* 1981;29:28-34.

Chen J, Normand ST. Myocardial infarction and quality of care. *Can Med Assoc J.* 2008;179:875-876.

Chobianm AV, Bakris GL, Black HR, et al. The National High Blood Pressure Education Program Coordinating Committee. The Seventh Report of the Joint National Committee on Prevention, Detection, Evaluation, and Treatment of High Blood Pressure. *J Am Med Assoc.* 2003;289:2560-2572.

Clark CE, Smith LF, Taylor RS, Cambell JL. Nurse led interventions to improve control of blood pressure in people with hypertension: systemic review meta-analysis. *Br J Med.* 2010;341:c3995.

Frasure-Smith N, Lesperance F, Prince RH, et al. Randomised trial of home-based psychosocial nursing intervention for patients recovering from myocardial infarction. *Lancet.* 1997;350:473-479.

Ghezeljeh TN, Momtahen M, Tessma MK, Nikravesh MY, Ekman I, Emami A. Gender specific variations in the description, intensity and location of angina pectoris: a cross-sectional study. *Int J Nurs Stud.* 2010;47:965.

Hardin SR, Steele JR. Atrial fibrillation among older adults: pathophysiology, symptoms, and treatment. *J Gerontol Nurs.* 2008;34:26-33.

Ignatavicius D, Workman ML. *Medical-Surgical Nursing: Patient-Centered Collaborative Care.* 7th ed. St Louis, MO: Elsevier; 2013.

Juenger J, Schellberg D, Kraemer S, et al. Health related quality of life in patients with congestive heart failure: comparison with other chronic diseases and relation to functional variables. *Heart.* 2002;87:235-241.

Koenig HG. Depression outcome in in-patients with congestive heart failure. *Arch Intern Med.* 2006;166:991-996.

Meghani SH, Becker D. Beta-blockers: a new therapy in congestive heart failure. *Am J Crit Care.* 2001;10:417-427.

Newton JL. Angina pectoris: a cry from the heart. *Nursing.* 1998;28:58-60.

Petty GW, Khandheria BK, Whisnant JP, Sicks JD, O'Fallon WM, Wiebers DO. Predictors of cerebrovascular events and death among patients with valvular heart disease: a population-based study. *Stroke.* 2000;31:2628-2635.

Porth CM. *Essentials of Pathophysiology.* 3rd ed. Philadelphia, PA: Lippincott Williams & Wilkins; 2011.

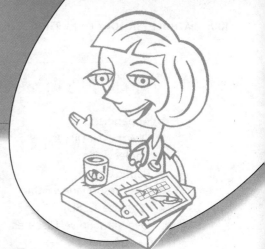

chapter 4

Gastrointestinal System

LEARNING OBJECTIVES

At the end of this chapter, the reader/student will be able to:

- Describe the physiology of the entire gastrointestinal system
- Compare the pathophysiology of appendicitis, diverticular disease, cholecystitis, peptic ulcers, gastroesophageal reflux disease, inflammatory bowel disorders, and liver disease
- Discuss nursing management of gastrointestinal disorders
- Differentiate among the surgical techniques and other treatments for GI problems

KEY WORDS

Appendicitis
Diverticular Disease
Cholecystitis
Peptic Ulcers
Gastroesophageal Reflux
  Disease (GERD)
Overview: Bowel Diseases

Ulcerative Colitis
Crohn's Disease
Overview: Liver Diseases
Cirrhosis
Hepatitis
Liver Failure

Introduction

The gastrointestinal (GI) system can be broken into portions, each of which has a particular function. The upper portion consists of the mouth, esophagus, stomach, and the duodenum and aids in ingestion and digestion of food. The lower GI tract is composed of the small and large intestines, the rectum, and anus. The organs that also play a part in the digestive process are the biliary system and the exocrine pancreas. The main functions of the gastrointestinal system are to convert ingested foods and liquids into a form that can be utilized by the cells of the body and to store and excrete the products of the digestive process. The mouth is where the food is chewed and mixed with saliva, which contains the enzyme ptyalin secreted by the parotid gland. The esophagus is a hollow tube that connects the mouth and the stomach and lies behind the trachea and it moves the food from the mouth by peristalsis to the stomach after swallowing. There is a sphincter at each end and both are closed during the swallowing process. The sphincters help prevent the reflux of acidic gastric contents. The stomach is located in the upper left abdomen and left of the liver and to the right of the spleen. The primary function of the stomach is to store the food and partially digest it. Pepsin is secreted in the stomach, and the stomach must be acidic for this enzyme to digest proteins. The gastric glands secrete a large quantity of hydrochloric acid, which is necessary for protein digestion but also protects the stomach by destroying any ingested microorganisms. The intrinsic factor is also secreted, which is essential for the absorption of vitamin B_{12}. The gallbladder is an organ that lies below the liver, and the major function is to store and concentrate the bile, which is formed in the liver. The bile is excreted into the common bile duct. The duct passes behind the pancreas and via the pancreatic duct empties into the duodenum. Sphincters regulate the flow of bile. The sphincter of Oddi regulates the flow into the duodenum, and a second sphincter regulates the flow of bile in the common bile duct. The pancreas secretes the enzyme trypsin, which breaks down protein; amylase, which breaks down starch; and lipase, which changes fats into glycerol and fatty acids. The small intestine is where the last stage of digestion occurs of proteins and it is where the proteins, fats, and complex carbohydrates are broken down by the bile and pancreatic enzymes so that they can be absorbed by the millions of villi in the small intestine, providing nutrients to the body. Absorption is accomplished by slow circular contractions and by diffusion or active transport, and then the leftover products (chyme) are propelled to the large colon. The large intestine's main function is to absorb water and electrolytes from the chyme and store the food waste until defecation, through the anus.

Appendicitis

The vermiform appendix is a small fingerlike projection attached to the cecum (a blind pouch that forms the first portion of the large intestine). Appendicitis occurs when there is an obstruction of the appendix, commonly caused by a fecalith (hardened stool), which causes inflammation. Other rarer causes can be foreign body or a neoplasm. It is the most common abdominal surgical emergency and affects about 10% of the population aged 10–30 years. The obstruction leads to increased abdominal pressure, congestion, and infection. If an inflamed appendix is left untreated, gangrene and perforation (rupture) will occur within 36 hours. Children who perforate may develop generalized peritonitis, which may result in mortality (Figure 4–1).

Clinical Manifestations

Fever, tachycardia, right lower quadrant tenderness, and maximal tenderness at McBurney point (halfway between the umbilicus and the anterior spine of the ileum) is the classic sign. Pain starts in the epigastric or umbilical region and then localizes in the right lower quadrant; pain may be accompanied by anorexia or vomiting. There is rebound tenderness and the person may lie on his or her side or back with the knees flexed.

Diagnostic Tests

Physical examination including a positive obturator sign (pain with internal rotation of flexed right thigh); a complete blood count (CBC) will show

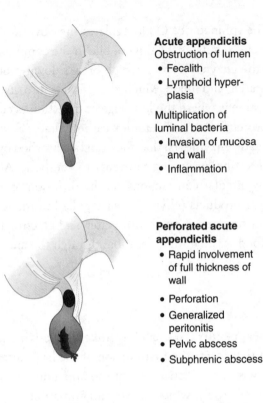

Acute appendicitis
Obstruction of lumen
- Fecalith
- Lymphoid hyper-
  plasia

Multiplication of
luminal bacteria
- Invasion of mucosa
  and wall
- Inflammation

**Perforated acute
appendicitis**
- Rapid involvement
  of full thickness of
  wall
- Perforation
- Generalized
  peritonitis
- Pelvic abscess
- Subphrenic abscess

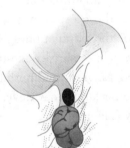

**Localized peritoneal
involvement**
- Inflammatory mass,
  or "phlegmon"
- Suppuration
- Appendiceal
  abscess
- Necrosis of
  appendix
- Gangrenous
  appendicitis

FIGURE 4–1 • Pathogenesis and complications of acute appendicitis. (Reproduced with permission from Chandrasoma P, et al. *Concise Pathology*. 3rd ed. New York: McGraw-Hill; 1997, figure 39-11.)

leukocytosis with white blood cells >10,000/mm^3; urinalysis may show hematuria or pyuria; ultrasonography or computed tomographic (CT) scan is the choice to diagnose. Also perform a human chorionic gonadotropin (hCG) test on a female to rule out pregnancy or ectopic pregnancy.

Treatment

Surgical treatment of an infected appendix is surgery. In some cases, antibiotics will be given intravenously to control the infection prior to surgery. Appendectomy is most often removed through a laparoscope today, leading to decreased hospital length of stay and reduced healing time.

Nursing Interventions and Complications

During the diagnostic period, the nurse must keep the patient as comfortable as possible, reduce anxiety, prepare the person for surgery, keep him or her on bed rest and give nothing by mouth (NPO), maintain intravenous (IV) fluids and electrolyte replacement, monitor lab values, and explain to the patient why pain medication may be withheld to avoid masking any critical changes. The nurse must closely monitor the patient for any signs of perforation, which can occur in 20% of patients whose pain has persisted for more than 36 hours, monitor temperature, and changes in pain. After the surgery, the nurse continues to monitor all vital signs and alleviate pain.

> **CLINICAL ALERT**
>
> *Include a question on the nursing history about constipation or difficulty passing stools in the differential diagnosis of potential appendicitis. Appendicitis must be diagnosed rapidly and treated because the potential for rupture and peritonitis usually occurs 36 hours after initial pain and symptoms begin. A quick diagnosis is imperative for early surgical intervention.*

Diverticular Disease

Diverticula are outpouchings or bulging sacs in the gastrointestinal wall. The wall pushes the mucous lining through the muscle. Diverticula can vary in size from a few millimeters to several centimeters. Although they can occur anywhere in the GI tract, 90%–95% are found in the sigmoid colon. The reason for this is that the colon has high pressure inside the lumen, and hard stool increases the pressure. Diverticula can be asymptomatic or cause some pain, which can be thought to be a case of irritable bowel syndrome, fecal impaction, gallbladder disease, appendicitis, or in female patients, ectopic pregnancy. In asymptomatic patients who may have other issues requiring a barium enema, diverticulosis is often found. The occurrence of diverticulosisis is usually seen in patients older than age 40 years and increases with advancing age. Risk factors include obesity, low-fiber diet, sedentary lifestyle, and the number of diverticula in the colon. Both men and women are equally affected by this disease. At any point of time, those with diverticulum (pouches in the mucosal lining) may progress to *diverticulitis*. Diverticulitis occurs when undigested food such as nuts or popcorn get stuck in the pouches and bacteria build up, which results in infection in the pouch or pouches. Most patients are managed medically based on the symptoms they experience and their history until the acute symptoms resolve, and then a colonoscopy and CT scan is performed for definitive diagnosis.

Clinical Manifestations

Diverticulitis causes pain that is mild to moderate because of inflammation from the infection, which is usually felt in the left lower quadrant. Other symptoms include constipation or loose stools, abdominal distention, and low-grade fever from the infection; nausea and vomiting are common. In severe diverticulitis, peritonitis may develop or there may be a large undrainable abscess that requires immediate surgery and removal of the diseased section of the colon.

Diagnostic Tests

CT scan of the abdomen; colonoscopy to rule out other diseases and determine the extent of the disease; CBC, which may be normal but if the patient is bleeding from the disease, the hemoglobin level may be low; and there may be blood in the stool, so a stool guaiac test should be done. Further, blood culture (would be positive if it is a case of generalized peritonitis), urine culture, and sensitivity testing (potential fistula postsurgically) should be performed.

Treatment

Medical management includes broad-spectrum antibiotics such as amoxicillin and clavulanate K, or metronidazole plus ciprofloxacin, and keeping the patient on a clear liquid diet. Patients who experience increasing pain, fever, or an inability to tolerate oral fluids require hospitalization, where they are kept NPO and IV antibiotics are administered. Those who do not improve within 72 hours of hospitalization should have a repeat abdominal CT, and patients with a localized abscess may need to have a catheter inserted to drain the abscess.

Nursing Interventions and Complications

During the acute phase when the patient is hospitalized, the nurse should be supportive and maintain patient comfort. The nurse must monitor electrolytes and lab values, maintain the IV site, and administer antibiotics, while assessing the patient frequently for signs of complication or increased pain. Patient education by the nurse in an outpatient setting and caring for asymptomatic diverticular disease include instructing on the importance of a high-fiber diet, exercise, weight loss, and prevention of constipation. The surgical patient requires close monitoring for signs of postoperative infection, should be encouraged to continue coughing and deep breathing and to maintain a semi-Fowler position, in addition to maintaining nasogastric (NG) tube functioning. The nurse needs to provide emotional care to the patient as in this situation anxiety is increased. The patient and family should be taught about the disease process and the nurse should support and encourage the patient and family. The overall treatment and any tests being done should be explained by the nurse, and the family should be informed of the routine and care of the patient when he or she is discharged home. The patient with peritonitis or a large abscess is very ill. The nurse should also be aware that fistula formation may occur that can involve the bladder, ureter, uterus, or the abdominal wall and the nurse should carefully assess the patient for this postsurgically.

CLINICAL ALERT

Perforation of a diverticulum may result in an intraabdominal infection or generalized peritonitis. Fistula formation may form and involve the bladder, ureter, vagina, uterus, bowel, and abdominal wall. Diverticulitis may constrict the colon, resulting in a partial or complete obstruction. Nurses must assess the patient for signs of infection and abdominal rigidity. Fistula formation should be suspected when a patient complains of other structures around the colon.

Cholecystitis

The gallbladder is a pear-shaped sac that lies attached underneath the liver. The major function is to store and concentrate the bile that is formed in the liver. The liver excretes bile into the hepatic ducts, which unite and form the common bile duct. The common bile duct passes behind the pancreas and is joined by the pancreatic duct, and the bile passes into the duodenum. Sphincters control the flow of bile in the common bile duct. When the sphincter is closed, the bile moves back to the gallbladder, which is responsible for concentrating the bile. Bile helps in the digestion and absorption of fats. When the gallbladder becomes inflamed because of an obstruction such as a gallstone or tumor, cholecystitis develops. Gallstones result when there is a change and composition of bile from the liver such as a high concentration of cholesterol, calcium, or bilirubin, which precipitate to form stones. The stones can lodge in the common bile duct, which can block the flow of bile into the duodenum. The narrowing and swelling may cause irritation to the common bile duct as well. Certain conditions such as obesity, age (older than 40 years), estrogen imbalance, and heredity are factors that may contribute to the development of gallstones. Both women and men can develop these biliary calculi, but obese women have a higher incidence. Gallstones occur in approximately 20% of the population. The gallbladder can become edematous and infection with fever and chill occurs. Medical management is to treat the infection, and then intervene surgically to remove the gallbladder. Today the gallbladder can be removed by laparoscopic surgery, which decreases the risks of surgery and decreases the hospital stay. People can live without a gallbladder because the liver can excrete bile directly into the duodenum.

Clinical Manifestations

Acute inflammation due to a gallstone can result in severe colicky pain felt in the right upper quadrant and through the back, which is made worse by eating fatty foods. Patients may experience nausea, vomiting, mildly elevated liver function tests, and signs of infection. Complications can occur depending where the obstruction is, such as pancreatitis, or gangrene if the blood supply is cut off. Some people have no symptoms at all and may find they have gallstones when having a sonogram or x-ray for some other issue.

Diagnostic Tests

Ultrasonography is one of the best tests to detect gallstones 97%–98% of the time. A CT scan can detect stones in the distal common bile duct. Lab test for liver function; endoscopic retrograde cholangiopancreatography (ERCP) is an invasive test and is used when noninvasive tests cannot diagnose the problem. Magnetic resonance imaging (MRI) is sensitive 90% of time.

Treatment

Acute cholecystitis may be treated conservatively by withholding any oral feedings and giving IV antibiotics and pain medication. If symptoms continue to persist, surgical intervention of removal of the gallbladder (cholecystectomy) is done. This procedure is usually done via a laparoscope. If there is evidence of gangrene of the gallbladder, immediate surgery is performed.

Nursing Implications and Complications

Symptomatic patients have a slightly increased mortality risk and a modest chance of complications. Nurses need to inform patients of the therapeutic options. Nurses explain the diagnostic tests the patient is to have, and administers ordered antibiotics if there is infection in the gallbladder prior to surgery. Nurses keep the patients on a nothing-by-mouth (NPO) diet; monitor lab values such as liver enzymes and amylase, and assess for pain both pre- and postoperatively. The nurse cares for the T-tube for drainage if the stone was in the common bile duct as well as assess for any signs of complications. If the nurse is in the community setting, education regarding weight reduction for obese patients and decreasing cholesterol and fatty foods in their diet, as well as increasing exercise, may prevent some patients from developing gallstones, thereby preventing surgery.

> **CLINICAL ALERT**
>
> *If a stone becomes lodged in the common bile duct, there is an increased risk of complications and death. Nurses must assess the patient for sepsis, gangrene, and jaundice, which can occur if the common bile duct is blocked.*

Peptic Ulcers

Peptic ulcers are lesions found in the lining of the duodenum, the lower end of the esophagus, or the stomach, which are areas exposed to gastric acid and pepsin. These ulcers occur in areas that are thought to be particularly vulnerable to the effects of acid, pepsin, bile, and pancreatic enzymes. This disease continues to be a major source of morbidity and affects about 10% and 5% of women in their lifetimes. Although the mechanism of how an ulcer is formed remains incompletely understood, the process seems to involve acid production, pepsin secretion, and *Helicobacter pylori* infection. Excess acid production is the main explanation of duodenal ulcers. Some patients with duodenal ulcer demonstrate rapid gastric emptying, which raises the acid exposure of the proximal duodenum. Aspirin and nonsteroidal antiinflammatory drugs (NSAIDs) taken over a long period of time are capable of producing a deep gastric ulcer. Infection with *H. pylori* has emerged as a very important cause of duodenal ulcer in 95%–99% of the cases. Other causes, for example, psychological issues such as stress, smoking and alcohol use, dietary issues such as coffee drinking, and use of glucocorticosteroid and heredity have been thought to increase one's susceptibility to peptic ulcers.

Clinical Manifestations

Some patients may present with pain, bleeding, nausea, anorexia, and obstruction, but others may be symptom-free. Twenty percent of patients with ulcer complications such as bleeding have no symptoms leading up to the bleeding episode. Epigastric pain (dyspepsia) is described as a gnawing, dull, aching pain or "hunger like" sensation. Approximately 50% of those with symptoms are relieved by antacids or food. Most ulcers cause nocturnal pain, which awakens the patient. Most patients have symptom-free periods lasting up to several weeks to months. Gastric ulcer pain is more likely to be worse with meals and radiates from the epigastrium to the back. The pain may be dull, gnawing, or burning in quality. There may be complaints of indigestion, vomiting, loss of appetite, or weight loss.

Diagnostic Tests

Lab tests for CBC with differential, fecal occult blood testing, *H. pylori* testing (urea breath test), serum amylase (suggests ulcer penetration into the pancreas), upper endoscopy, and barium or Gastrografin contrast radiography, when endoscopy is unsuitable or not feasible.

Treatment

Use of proton pump inhibitors that bind the acid-secreting enzyme is the most common treatment. If *H. pylori* is found, treatment with combination antibiotics such as clarithromycin and amoxicillin is followed. Avoid the use of aspirin or NSAIDs. With treatment, most ulcers are healed in 8 weeks.

Nursing Interventions and Complications

Acid suppression drugs are given and explained to the patient such as proton pump inhibitors (PPI). If *H. pylori* infection is diagnosed, the nurse either treats the patient with antibiotics or explains to the patient how to take the antibiotics, such that no ethanol alcohol (EtOH) is consumed while taking metronidazole. The nurse monitors the lab values, as the patient may have an ulcer that is bleeding causing anemia, heme-positive stool, or vomiting of blood. Complications could be perforation, hemorrhage, or risk of gastric adenocarcinoma, which is increased in patients infected with *H. pylori*. The nurse will also counsel the patient on smoking cessation and ways to cope with stress more effectively.

> **CLINICAL ALERT**
>
> *Upper gastrointestinal bleeding is clinically significant in approximately 10% of ulcer patients. Those with severe bleeding may die, especially elderly patients or those with comorbid medical problems. Mortality is higher in patients with persistent hypotension, shock, bright red blood in the vomitus, or severe coagulopathy. Nurses must be alert to changes in CBC and assess patients with ulcer disease for obvious or occult bleeding.*

Gastroesophageal Reflux Disease (GERD)

Reflux of gastroduodenal contents into the esophagus, larynx, or lungs with or without causing inflammation. Most cases of GERD are attributed to loss of the normal pressure gradient between the lower esophageal sphincter (LES) and the stomach. The LES is a high-pressure zone of smooth muscle that straddles the diaphragm and is the major component of the antireflux barrier. The major symptom, heartburn, is the most common disorder of the esophagus, and the major indication for antacid consumption. It is estimated that 44% of Americans experience heartburn at least once every month. Transient relaxation of the LES accounts for nearly all episodes of reflux in healthy subjects and about 65% of episodes in patients with GERD. Problems that require further investigation are esophageal symptoms that are not responding to medical treatments such as the prescription antacids such as proton pump inhibitors (e.g., omeprazole), or H2 antagonists (e.g., cimetidine). All patients with persistent reflux symptoms or frequent relapses, even if they are on medications, should have endoscopy to identify possible esophagitis or complications that may require biopsies to exclude malignancies. The presence of odynophagia (pain with swallowing) usually is associated with ulcerative esophagitis. Foods that can contribute to GERD are high-fat, citrus, or spicy foods; chocolate; peppermint; and onions. Some other factors that can contribute to people having GERD are obesity, delayed gastric emptying, positional changes such as bending, or ineffective peristalsis. Smoking and use of alcohol or caffeine are risk factors for GERD. Barrett esophagus is a condition where there is a change from squamous epithelium in the distal esophagus to metaplastic columnar epithelium, which represents chronic exposure of the esophagus to stomach acid. Barrett esophagus causes pathologic changes that occur after having GERD for many years and is occasionally followed by adenocarcinoma. If all treatment for GERD is ineffective and a patient continues to have severe symptoms, laparoscopic surgery may be an option. During the surgery, an attempt to maintain a segment of the tubular esophagus below the diaphragm and wrapping the stomach around the distal end of the esophagus to produce an increased LES pressure is the goal. The long-term results from having the surgery is about 80%.

Clinical Manifestations

Symptoms include heartburn (retrosternal burning) that usually occurs 30–60 minutes after a meal, regurgitation of digested food, angina-like chest pain, abdominal pain, hoarseness, dysphagia (many cases a result of erosive esophagitis), bronchospasm, aspiration of food (which could lead to aspiration pneumonia), chronic cough, sour taste in mouth, and loss of dental enamel. Atypical symptoms when the esophagus is damaged due to the acid are asthma, chromic laryngitis, and sore throat.

Diagnostic Tests

Twenty-four-hour pH monitoring is the most important test as well as the patient keeping a record of the number of reflux episodes that occur when the patient is upright; another test is an esophageal manometry that records the pressure of the LES. A barium swallow test may be done, and endoscopy is recommended in the older patient who continues to have symptoms after 4 weeks of treatment.

Treatment

Uncomplicated GERD are treated with a proton pump inhibitor for 4–8 weeks. Patient must be taught to eat smaller meals and eliminate acidic foods such as citrus, tomatoes, spicy foods, alcohol, and tobacco. Complicated cases involving the esophagus may require surgery to either stretch the esophagus if strictures are present to remove the damaged part of the esophagus caused by the gastric reflux.

Nursing Interventions and Complications

Nurses educate patients with GERD about dietary agents that increase their symptoms, such as caffeine, alcohol, chocolate, and spicy foods and to eat small meals and to avoid lying down after meals. Nurses also counsel the patients to stop smoking and refer them to centers to help with smoking cessation as well as encourage patients to lose weight. Nurses monitor the patients for complications such as peptic strictures in which mucosal damage is caused by constant erosion and being healed again produces scar tissue. This can progress to dysphagia and aspiration pneumonia. Nurses must also monitor the CBC to assess for bleeding from the mucosal ulcer or corrosive esophagitis. Nurses also explain all the diagnostic tests that the patient may need as well as prepare the patient for surgery if it is required.

> **CLINICAL ALERT**
>
> *GERD, which leads to esophageal changes, may result in Barrett esophagus where the cells undergo changes in which the most serious complication is esophageal carcinoma. Strictures in the esophagus occur in about 5% of patients. Solid food dysphagia occurs. Dilation of the esophagus is the only treatment. Nurses must assess symptoms and treat GERD early and assess the patient frequently to limit the severe consequences of the disease.*

Overview: Bowel Diseases

There are several bowel diseases all of which cause pain, change in bowel functioning, and alteration in quality of life. Irritable bowel syndrome (IBS) is a functional disorder (a term describing a symptom or group of symptoms for which no organic disease can be found). It has also been called spastic colon as there are varying degrees of pain associated with IBS and there can be symptoms of constipation and/or diarrhea, bloating, passage of mucus, and feeling of bloating. It is one of the most common gastrointestinal disorders and accounts for 50% of the visits to see a gastroenterologist. Women are diagnosed with IBS 2:1 more times than men. The diagnosis of IBS is usually made from the symptoms experienced and when tests such as a sigmoidoscopy or colonoscopy prove negative for any pathologic bowel change. Pharmacologic agents do not treat IBS well, and often antispasmodics with an anticholinergic effect work best. There has been correlation of those under stress having more bouts of IBS attacks. The more serious bowel diseases with noted pathology and lifelong suffering are ulcerative colitis and Crohn's disease, which will be discussed in detail.

Ulcerative Colitis

This is an inflammatory disease in which extensive areas of the walls in the large intestine become inflamed, edematous, and ulcerated. The mucosa is very fragile and bleeds spontaneously or in response to minimal trauma. The motility of ulcerated colon is very high and colon secretions are increased greatly, thereby causing repeated diarrheal bowel movements, which are often bloody. The pattern of ulceration begins in the rectum and extends proximally in a continuous manner and can involve the entire colon. The disease is usually confined to the rectosigmoid in most patients and less than 20% have involvement in the entire colon. This is a chronic disease that can be characterized by periods of exacerbation and remission. The etiology of ulcerative colitis is unknown but some hypotheses include allergies to certain foods, and abnormal immune response to bacteria or self-antigens. Those with severe exacerbations are treated with hydrocortisone, but those taking hydrocortisone on and off for long periods of time gain weight, experience bone loss, have increased infections, and may have increased glucose levels. They may be treated long term with oral sulfasalazine to help prevent exacerbations. These drugs have side effects and must be monitored for liver and renal function as well as CBC. Those with colitis may also have common associated conditions such as pyoderma gangrenosum (ulcerating skin disease in which the skin in infiltrated with neutrophils), erythema nodosum (a tender red nodular rash on shins), arthritic condition of large joints, or thromboembolic disease. This disease can greatly alter the patient's quality of life because when severe exacerbations occur one cannot go to work or function well as most of the day is spent in pain with diarrhea, and further discomfort if they suffer from any of the associated conditions mentioned. Up to 25% of patients with extensive UC ultimately require colectomy (removal of part of the colon).

Clinical Manifestations

Lower abdominal pain, diarrhea, blood with stools, fever, associated skin manifestations, rectal urgency, tenesmus (spasmodic contraction of the anus with pain and persistent desire to empty bowel), anorexia, fatigue, and malaise, and some patients experience arthralgias and arthritis.

Diagnostic Tests

Barium enema test, sigmoidoscopy, colonoscopy (during the disease, those with ulcerative colitis undergo many colonoscopies to assess progression of disease and biopsy to ensure that the eroded areas have not turned malignant). Lab tests done are CBC, C-reactive protein (CRP), sedimentation rate, serum albumin, electrolytes, and liver function tests.

Treatment

Treatment is aimed at stopping the acute attack and prevention of recurrent attacks. The treatment depends on the extent of colonic involvement and how severe the illness is. Mild to moderate disease is treated with drugs such as mesalamine, balsalazide, and sulfasalazine. If the patient does not improve in 6–8 weeks, corticosteroids are added. If patients continue to have exacerbations, an immunomodulating agent may be added but the risks from chronic immunosuppression must be weighed carefully. As a last resort, surgery to remove the affected part of the colon is removed. Those with ulcerative colitis continue to have periods of acute attacks.

Nursing Interventions and Complications

If the patient is hospitalized or the nurse is providing home care, assessment for fluid volume deficit due to diarrhea and blood loss must be assessed. Nurses should educate the patient on the negative association with smoking and colitis. Assess the patient for any of the associated complications. Assess lab data for abnormalities, with special attention to sodium, potassium, albumin, bicarbonate, and calcium. Provide emotional support as patients who suffer from this chronic disorder may be anxious or depressed. Assess for possible perforation due to friability of the colon, and if the patient requires surgery provide pre- and postoperative care as well as educate the patients about the tests required and what to expect from the surgery.

> ## CLINICAL ALERT
>
> *Patients with severe ulcerative colitis may have more than 6–10 bloody stools per day resulting in severe anemia, impaired nutrition with hypoalbuminemia. Fulminant colitis can occur in severe disease in which symptoms rapidly worsen with signs of toxicity. Patients must be monitored and assessed frequently.*

Crohn's Disease

This is a nonspecific, chronic inflammatory disease that commonly affects the distal ileum and the proximal colon. The mucosa is chronically inflamed and the submucosa is thickened by the dense fibrous tissue. The areas of strictures that are thickened may cause narrowing and can cause perforations leading to fistula formation that could connect with the bladder, vagina, or other segment of the bowel. These strictures that form can also make it impossible to pass an endoscope to view the disease and monitor the progression. Crohn's disease may involve multiple regions in the intestine, and in between these areas there may be normal tissue. It can occur at any age but predominantly occurs between the ages 15 and 25, with another peak at age 55–65. Fifteen percent of the patients who have Crohn's disease have a first-degree relative with the disease. There is also a 2%–4% increase in Crohn's disease in the Ashkenazi Jewish population. The etiology is a combination of genetic, environmental factors, and immunologic abnormalities. In Crohn's disease, the role of inflammatory mediators play a role as the T-helper cells in the bowel mucosa appear to produce an increased amount of tumor necrosis factor (TNF), factor-α. Infusion of monoclonal antibodies against these cytokines (1 or more than 100 distinct proteins produced primarily by white blood cells), can produce remission in otherwise very difficult cases of Crohn's disease. This disease causes weight loss because of its effect on the small intestine. Fat-soluble vitamins such as A, D, E, and K may be poorly absorbed. They may require multiple hospitalizations because of the severity of the symptoms. Surgery may be required for failure of medical management, total or recurrent intestinal obstruction, perforation, hemorrhage, abscess formation, symptomatic fistula, or failure of an ostomy to function. Even with surgery for resection, there is often relapse of the disease. Patients with Crohn's disease are at an increased risk of developing colon cancer (Figure 4–2).

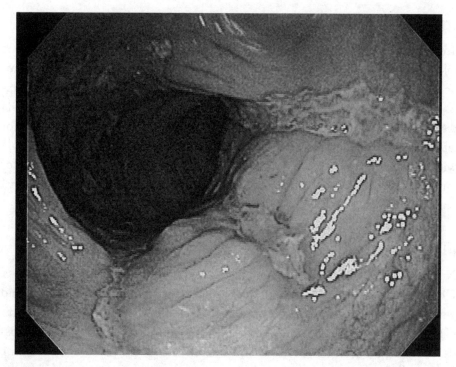

FIGURE 4–2 • Crohn's colitis with deep longitudinal ulcers and normal appearing tissue in between. The biopsies that showed normal tissue between the ulcers clinched the diagnosis for Crohn's disease. Ulcerative colitis is diffuse whereas Crohn's disease often skips areas as seen in this patients colon. (Reproduced with permission from Usatine RP, et al. *The Color Atlas of Family Medicine*. New York: McGraw-Hill; 2009, figure 62-5. Courtesy of Marvin Derezin, MD.)

Clinical Manifestations

Intermittent attacks of diarrhea and may be bloody fecal urgency, fever, abdominal pain, anorexia, weight loss, fistula formation, intestinal obstruction, arthritis, skin disorders (nonspecific rashes, erythema nodosum, and pyoderma gangrenosum [see explanation in Ulcerative Colitis section for the latter two]), malaise, increased incidence of gallstones, and a palpable tender mass that represents thickened inflamed loops of intestine.

Diagnostic Tests

Lab test for anemia CBC with differential, sedimentation rate, serum albumin levels, electrolytes, vitamin B_{12}, perinuclear antineutrophil cytoplasmic antibody (p-ANCA) that is elevated in Crohn's disease, C-reactive protein, barium enema, CT scans, colonoscopy, biopsy of mucosa, esophagogastroduodenoscopy (EGD, which allows direct visualization).

Treatment

Treatment is prednisone to treat the inflammation, sulfasalazine or mesalamine taken everyday, and methotrexate weekly is given to achieve remission. Immunomodulators are used if corticosteroids fail. Anti-TNF therapy such as infliximab and adalimumab are used for treatment in severe cases including fistula disease. Patients may be on maintenance therapy and must be monitored for labs as Anti-TNF may increase the risk of lymphoma. Fifty percent of people with Crohn's disease will require at least one surgical procedure because of intraabdominal abscess, massive bleeding, perianal fistulas, or intestinal obstruction.

Nursing Implications and Complications

Nurses must monitor nutrition and assess subcutaneous fat and muscle mass. Observe amount and character of diarrhea, teach the patient about illness and what to know about complications and whom to call, and refer to a Crohn's disease support group. Monitor lab values and administer medication for disease looking for allergic reactions and side effects. If patient is not absorbing foods well, decrease the fat in the diet; also make sure patient stops smoking by referring to a smoking cessation group, as smoking exacerbates the disease. Provide emotional support for this chronic severe illness. If patient requires surgery, provide pre- and postoperative care. Include the family in the plan of this chronic disease.

> **CLINICAL ALERT**
>
> *Crohn's disease can cause intestinal obstruction by narrowing of the small bowel as a result of continued inflammation, fistulas can penetrate through the bowel to adjacent structures and abscess can cause fever, chills, and recurrent infections. Perianal disease can also occur. Because Crohn's disease increases the risk for colon cancer, nurses must teach the patient that frequent colonoscopy is necessary. Nurses must monitor and assess these patients for all these complications.*

Overview: Liver Diseases

The liver is the largest and one of the most complex organs in the body and it is located below the diaphragm in the upper quadrant of the abdomen. It receives its blood from two sources, as oxygenated blood under high pressure comes from the hepatic artery and the rest comes via the portal vein, and brings blood rich in nutrients under loss of pressure from the stomach, intestines, spleen, and pancreas. These sources mix as they begin to flow through the liver and collect in the left and right hepatic veins, which then drain into the inferior vena cava. It is one of the most complex organs in the body. There is a ligament called the falciform that divides the liver into the right and left lobes and provides attachment to the anterior abdominal wall. The liver extends from the fifth intercostal space to up and under the ribs making it 4–8 cm in height at the midsternal line and 6–12 cm in height at the midclavicular line. The functional unit of the liver is the lobules, and each lobule consists of cellular plates that empty into the bile ducts. The terminal bile ducts join to form the hepatic duct, which joins with the cystic duct of the gallbladder to form the common bile duct. The liver can be thought of as a waste disposal unit. The liver performs many functions. The liver converts fructose and galactose to glucose and removes excess glucose from the blood in response to insulin; it makes and stores glycogen, which can be reconverted to glucose when glucose levels fall; it breaks down phospholipids, triglycerides, and cholesterol; it manufactures bile to send to the gallbladder for use as needed; removes excess amino acids from the blood and converts them to other needed amino acids; the liver stores copper, vitamins including B_{12}; it synthesizes plasma proteins needed for blood clotting such as albumin (which hold water in the blood vessels), fibrinogen, and prothrombin; it digests bacteria and toxins to cleanse the blood; detoxifies substances such as urea from amino acid metabolism; and converts ammonia to urea for excretion. The liver can renew itself as cells can proliferate rapidly in response to injury and cell loss. Liver cells can be damaged by drugs, alcohol, chemicals, or viruses. Severe disease or chronic progressive disease can lead to permanent scarring and damage that make it impossible for the liver to regenerate. Injury or toxins can affect the release of bilirubin and the slow release can cause jaundice, which is yellowing of the body due to excessive bilirubin levels (Figures 4–3 and 4–4).

Cirrhosis

Cirrhosis is the end result of chronic liver disease. This is a chronic, progressive, irreversible damage to the liver that results in verycompromised liver function. It is the seventh leading cause of death in the United States and it affects approximately 11 million Americans. It is a disease mainly caused by

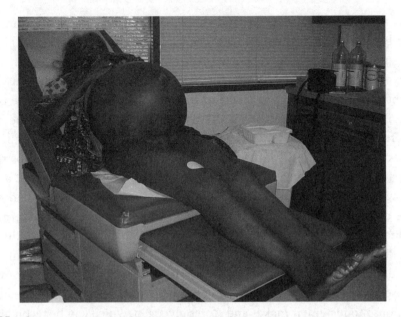

FIGURE 4–3 • Tense ascites in a woman with cirrhosis from heralcoholism. An umbilical hernia is also seen from the increased intra-abdominal pressure. (Reproduced with permission from Usatine RP, et al. *The Color Atlas of Family Medicine.* New York: McGraw-Hill; 2009, figure 58-5. Courtesy of Richard P. Usatine, MD.)

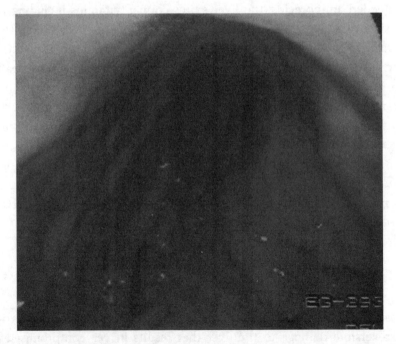

FIGURE 4–4 • Esophageal varices in the patient in Figure 4–5 secondary to her cirrhosis and portal hypertension. (Reproduced with permission from Usatine RP, et al. *The Color Atlas of Family Medicine.* New York: McGraw-Hill; 2009, figure 58-2. Courtesy of Javid Ghandehari, MD.)

chronic alcohol consumption. The liver is taxed so much that the damaged liver cells are replaced with thick, inflexible scar tissue. The scar tissue contracts and the organ shrinks, and this can produce a nodular, bumpy appearance that interferes with normal vascular and bile pathways. When the branches of the hepatic artery and portal vein are constricted by the scar tissue, it causes high pressure in the blood vessels leading to the liver and causes them to swell, and varices develop especially in the abdomen and esophagus. The organs that are connected to the liver's circulation such as the spleen, pancreas, and stomach swell as pressure rises. Even though some of the blood is to be shunted by collateral circulatory pathways, the veins in the systemic system cannot handle the high pressure and they dilate. Thus, varicosities are formed that can cause a slow bleed or they rupture and cause hemorrhage. In patients with cirrhosis, ascites develops because of (1) the high pressure within the obstructed portal system that forces fluids back up into the abdominal cavity and (2) the damaged liver cannot produce a sufficient supply of albumin that is necessary to maintain osmotic pressure and keep fluid in the capillaries so the fluid leaks out of the capillaries and leaks into the abdomen. Edema occurs, especially in the lower extremities. Jaundice occurs in these patients because of the liver's inability to move the bile and it builds in the liver and causes inflammation and necrosis and leaks into the bloodstream, causing jaundice. The changes in protein metabolism result in decreased production of protein clotting factors and muscle wasting. Severely damaged hepatic cells lose the ability to detoxify the blood and poisons accumulate, one of which is ammonia, and can produce neurologic symptoms such as confusion, disorientation, and hand tremor and involuntary jerky movements (asterixis). This is called encephalopathy. A bleed that may occur increases the protein level, or ingestion of protein can cause rapid encephalopathy, which can lead to infection, renal failure (also increasing proteins), and death is common. Because alcoholism is a widespread problem and many of those addicted to it do not want to stop and they continue to consume alcohol, they can die a slow painful death as liver failure occurs because of the chronic ingestion of the toxin. Those who are addicted to drugs, chronic ingestion of high doses of acetaminophen, and hepatitis can result in liver failure. If a person stops drinking ETOH before severe liver damage has occurred, the liver can repair itself and may live a longer life. The only medications that can be used just to alleviate some of the symptoms of severe disease is ursodiol to help to decrease bile salts, and propranolol to lower portal pressure; lactulose can be used for encephalopathy to induce at least three loose bowel movements a day to decrease ammonia levels (Figure 4–5).

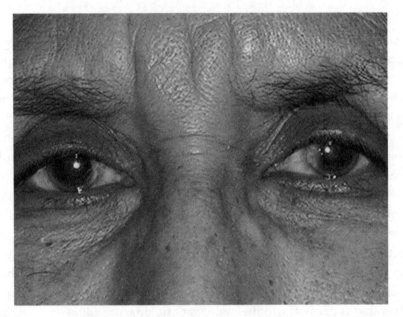

FIGURE 4–5 • Scleral icterus in a 64-year-old Hispanic woman with primary biliary cirrhosis. (Reproduced with permission from Usatine RP, et al. *The Color Atlas of Family Medicine.* New York: McGraw-Hill; 2009, figure 58-1. Courtesy of Javid Ghandehari, MD.)

Clinical Manifestations

Skin changes such as spider angiomata, jaundice (yellowing) of the sclera, ecchymoses, hepatomegaly, splenomegaly (from portal hypertension), fatigue, malaise, right upper quadrant pain, anorexia, muscle cramps, weight loss, central obesity, abdominal fluid wave (ascites), spider angioma on upper half of body, palmar erythema, asterixis (tremor and involuntary movements), mental changes, muscle wasting and weakness, epitaxies (nose bleeds), and pretibial or sacral edema.

Diagnostic Tests

Alanine aminotransferase (ALT), aspartame aminotransferase (AST), alkaline phosphatase (ALP), and γ-glutamyltranspeptidase (GGT) are those liver enzymes that would be elevated; decreased platelet count, low albumin and cholesterol levels, prolonged prothrombin time (PT), International Normalized Ratio (INR), and partial thromboplastin time (PTT). In progressive cirrhosis, there would be elevated blood urea nitrogen (BUN), ammonia, sodium, and potassium levels. An elevated α-fetoprotein level is used to screen for hepatocellular carcinoma. Tests include ultrasonography, Doppler study of hepatic/portal veins, MRI to clarify patency of blood vessels, liver biopsy, liver-spleen scan to diagnose portal hypertension, and endoscopy to rule out esophageal varices.

Treatment

Abstinence from alcohol should be stressed. Diet should contain adequate calories and in hepatic encephalopathy, protein should be limited; vitamin supplementation, in fluid retention sodium restriction; diagnostic paracentesis in new ascites; diuretic if fluid retention sodium restriction not adequate. A transjugular intrahepatic portosystemic shunt (TIPS) has shown benefit in the treatment of variceal bleeding. A stent is inserted between a branch of the hepatic vein and portal vein. The catheter is inserted in the jugular.

Nursing Implications and Complications

Nurses assess for nutrition and observe for anorexia, nausea, muscle wasting, and should weigh patient every day, assess fluid volume excess and monitor sodium, potassium, cholesterol, and all electrolytes, assess hepatojugular reflex, assess abdominal and overall body for edema, assess lungs for dyspnea, monitor blood pressure, assess mental function, assess skin integrity for turgor, presence of edema, ascites, and accumulation of bile salts on the skin; assess for bleeding as there is a high risk of bleeding, and monitor all clotting factors including vitamin K, provide emotional support without judgement as the patient may feel vulnerable and have a disturbed body image, and may verbalize his or her role in the self-destructive behavior that caused the illness causing suffering with all the complications of cirrhosis and facing potential death.

CLINICAL ALERT

Hepatic encephalopathy is when the central nervous system becomes disordered as a result of the liver failing to detoxify noxious agents such as ammonia. Lactulose can be given to decrease ammonia through frequent stool. There is low-grade cerebral edema and progresses from confusion to stupor and coma. Breathing becomes difficult because of increasing ascites. Bleeding from esophageal varices may result in hemorrhage and death.

Hepatitis

Viral and nonviral forms of hepatitis (inflammation of the liver) are more common than generally thought. There are more than 50,000 cases of viral hepatitis in the United States reported to the Centers for Disease Control and Prevention each year, although the actual number is thought to be up to 10 times as high. There are many viruses that cause hepatitis, and hepatitis B accounts for 30%–35% of the cases. Hepatitis A accounts for about 45%–50% of the cases and C for 15%–20%. There is also hepatitis D and E. Hepatitis A and E are self-limited and do not lead to chronic liver disease. Hepatitis B, C, and D can cause chronic hepatitis and cirrhosis. Hepatitis B and C can be complicated by hepatocellular carcinoma. Some people with these viruses progress to chronic infection whereas others become asymptomatic carriers of the virus. The ones that have chronic hepatitis are at an increased risk of developing cirrhosis and death. In most cases, acute viral hepatitis is a self-limiting illness where 85% of hospitalized patients and 95% of outpatients recover uneventfully in 3 months. The ways one contracts hepatitis A is from traveling to developing countries, employment in health care, household exposure to someone who has hepatitis, intimate exposure, especially male-with-male sex, institutionalized individuals, eating contaminated food or contact with someone with poor personal hygiene, or shellfish such as clams and mussels contaminated with hepatitis A virus (HAV). Hepatitis B is transmitted by exposure to blood and body fluids of infected people. Health care workers are at an increased risk of contracting hepatitis B through needle sticks or a splash with body fluids. Sexual transmission is an efficient mode of spreading the disease, as well as IV drug use. If a person is exposed to hepatitis B, prophylaxis can be initiated by giving immunoglobulin and hepatitis B vaccine. In the past, posttransfusion cases of hepatitis B resulted, but now there are sensitive screening methods to detect HBV as well as screening blood to prevent transfusion-transmitted AIDS. Treatments for the suppressions of viral replication of hepatitis B are interferon and other antiviral medications. Hepatitis D can be a superinfection or can be a coinfection with hepatitis B. Hepatitis E is spread from the fecal–oral route. Hepatitis C can be transmitted the same way as all the hepatitis viruses, which is sexual, exposure to infected body and fluids, organ transplant prior to 1992 before organs were screened for hepatitis, needle sticks, unsterile body piercing or tattoos, foreign travel, and people who have chronically high alanine aminotransferase (ALT) and aspartate aminotransferase (AST). There are vaccines for hepatitis A and hepatitis B (series of three vaccines).

Nonviral hepatitis can result from drugs/alcohol, industrial toxins, and plant poisons; health care workers are wary of adverse liver problems from mixing powder medications (e.g., chemotherapy).

There is also autoimmune hepatitis, which is an inflammatory disorder of the liver of unknown etiology and is characterized by hypergammaglobulinemia and autoantibodies. It occurs more often in females and has an abrupt onset, and one of its signs can be acute fulminant hepatic failure. To test for autoimmune hepatitis, autoantibodies with titers, antinuclear antibodies (ANAs), anti–smooth muscle antibodies (ASMAs), antibodies to liver/kidney microsomes (ALKM-1), and other tests can be performed.

Clinical Manifestations

Fever, malaise, nausea/vomiting, anorexia, jaundice/icterus, dark urine, pale stools, right upper quadrant pain, abdominal pain, splenomegaly, arthralgias, myalgias, pruritus, hepatomegaly, and infection in alcoholic hepatitis.

Diagnostic Tests

ALT/AST, bilirubin, alkaline phosphatase, PT, albumin, and ultrasonography may help diagnose ascites; contrast CT/MRI and liver biopsy can be performed for all hepatitis. Below are those specific to each type of hepatitis:

Hepatitis A: Anti-HAV immunoglobulin M, anti-HAV immunoglobulin G

Hepatitis B: serologic markers, hepatitis D (HDV), hepatitis Be antigen (HBeAg), screen for HIV, HCV, and immunity to HAV.

Hepatitis C: HCV RNA

Treatment

Bedrest only if symptoms of nausea and vomiting are bad. Strenuous exertion, alcohol, and hepatotoxic agents must be avoided. Medication given to avoid chronic hepatitis is Peginterferon. In many cases, complete recovery occurs, but 12% of acute liver failure is due to viral hepatitis.

Nursing Implications and Complications

Nurses should take a comprehensive health history and identify risks that may be associated with hepatitis or exposure to IV drug use, contaminated food, exposure to or sexual activity with one exposed to hepatitis. Educate all on preventing hepatitis A and B by getting vaccinated.

Monitor liver function tests, assess for jaundice (skin, sclera), hepatic enlargement, lymph node enlargement, right upper quadrant pain, petechiae, or bruises. Weigh patient every day, monitor temperature, food intake, fatigue, and assess for any increase of liver disease symptoms. Most patients recover from acute viral hepatitis, but chronic hepatitis may occur.

CLINICAL ALERT

Cirrhosis develops in 40% of those with chronic hepatitis B and even higher when coinfected with B and C. Patients with cirrhosis are at a higher risk of hepatocellular carcinoma. Nurses must educate patients on the risks involved in contracting hepatitis. Vaccines for hepatitis B and C are available.

Liver Failure

The term *liver failure* is used when the degree of liver necrosis affects more than 80%–90% of the liver, resulting in loss of liver function. It is the most dreaded outcome of any liver disorder. It is also termed fulminant hepatic failure. It is an uncommon condition in which a previously healthy person develops severe liver dysfunction with rapid-onset encephalopathy and/or bleeding. It is a highly complex syndrome that can arise in a few days or weeks, which causes about 75% of those with the disorder dying within days after the onset of symptoms. There is sudden massive necrosis of the liver cells; multiple organ failure involving the kidney, lungs, and circulatory system, which may be caused by the loss of hepatocyte function, some other cell mediators such as interleukin 1 (cytokine released by all nucleated cells and that modulates the liver as well as many other areas of the body), and tumor necrosis factor. Microvascular obstruction with some cellular debris from the damaged liver can impair tissue oxygenation and lead to lactic acidosis and circulatory collapse. Cerebral edema can occur from fluid overload, and the liver fails to manufacture the coagulation factors I, II, V, VII, IX, and X, which leads to bleeding. Patients with acute liver failure are also at a higher risk of developing infections. The causes of liver failure can be from hepatitis B, acetaminophen overdose (8–10 g in an adult or >150–200 mg/kg), some antibiotics, NSAIDs, anticoagulants, some herbal supplements (e.g., Kava Kava or ephedra), some viruses (e.g., Epstein-Barr, cytomegalovirus), toxins (e.g., wild mushrooms), autoimmune hepatitis, diseases of the veins of the liver leading to blockage, hepatic cancer (sixth most common cancer in the world), and primary biliary cirrhosis. The only treatment for acute liver failure is transplantation.

Clinical Manifestations

Encephalopathy caused by cerebral edema as a result of lack of oxygen (goes through stages from confusion to obtundation); bleeding anywhere, with attention to GI bleed; infection (respiratory, urinary); jaundice; itching; pain in right upper quadrant; kidney failure; dyspnea, ascites

Diagnostic Tests

Abdominal ultrasonography, Doppler study of hepatic veins, liver function test (ALT, AST), bilirubin, ammonia level, coagulation studies, CT/MRI, toxicology tests for drugs such as overdose of acetaminophen, renal function test (e.g., BUN, creatinine), albumin level, respiratory function test, liver biopsy, EGD (to assess for esophagogastric and gastric varices).

Treatment

Treatment is aimed toward correcting metabolic abnormalities such as coagulation defects, acid-base corrections, chronic kidney disease, hypoglycemia, and encephalopathy. Prophylactic antibiotics are given to decrease risk of infection. Early transfer to a liver transplantation center is essential for liver failure. Keep head of bed elevated to 30 degrees. Lactulose is administered for encephalopathy and mannitol can be given for cerebral edema. Patients waiting for transplant who have had an esophageal bleed may be put on a beta-blocker such as Inderal or Corgard, and ascites is treated with sodium restriction and a potassium-sparing diuretic such as Aldactone or a sulfonamide-derived loop diuretic such as Lasix.

Nursing Interventions and Complications

If an overdose of Tylenol is suspected, administer N-acetylcysteine (Mucomyst) after a gastric lavage; assess for any bleeding, provide nutrition with diet, with low or no protein, monitor respiratory function, and function, monitor lab values, assess for signs of decreased level of consciousness, assess for jaundice, monitor temperature, BP, heart rate and rhythm, provide education regarding liver transplant and its possible rejection, encourage patient to verbalize about fears about disease and prepare for death if donor not available in time. Ascites is treated with sodium restriction and a potassium-sparing diuretic such as Aldactone or a sulfonamide-derived loop diuretic such as Lasix. Complications such as bleeds or ascites must be managed first before transplantation can occur, which means patients with acute liver failure often die of the disease and complications before they receive a liver transplant.

CLINICAL ALERT

The mortality rate of fulminant hepatic failure with severe encephalopathy is as high as 80%. The outlook is extremely poor in patients younger than 10 and older than 40 years of age.

Acetaminophen toxicity is the most common cause of liver failure. Nursing must educate patients on the risks of taking large amounts of acetaminophen, which may result in a decreased number of those dying with liver failure.

CASE STUDY

MG is a Caucasian woman 53 years of age. She is 5' 4" and weighs 160 lbs. She has been suffering with a chronic GI condition for 15 years, which causes her severe lower quadrant pain and has frequent bloody stools. When she has a severe attack, she must stay home from work as she is in the bathroom frequently. She was being maintained on one previous medication, Asacol 800 mg three times a day, and now she is on Azulfidine 1000 mg three times a day. During her numerous attacks, she was treated with high doses of prednisone and has gained weight from all the prednisone and has developed osteoporosis and is taking Actonel 35 mg weekly. She has had numerous colonoscopies to monitor the disease. For the past 2 months, MG has been having upper right quadrant pain, which radiates into her back and she vomited once. The patient describes her pain as severe but it comes and goes. When she is questioned about the pain, it seems to occur after she has had ice cream or gravy with her meal, or when she eats out and has fried food. She has no other medical condition, but she smokes and walks her dog at night.

QUESTIONS

1. What condition has MG suffered from for 15 years?
2. Which changes in her lifestyle would you tell her to adopt and what referrals would you make?
3. What could her current symptoms suggest?
4. What diagnostic tests would be ordered for MG?
5. Which are some differential diagnoses that could cause similar symptoms?

Suggested Readings

Bhandari BM, Bayat H, Rothstein KD. Primary biliary cirrhosis. *Gastroenterol Clin N Am*. 2011;40:373-386.

Corall AH, Mulby AG. *Primary Care Medicine*. 4th ed. Philadelphia, PA: Lippincott Williams & Wilkins; 2000.

Cronin E. Prednisolone in the management of patients with Crohn's disease. *J Br Nurs*. 2009;19:1333-1336.

Dambro MR. *Griffith's 5 Minute Clinical Consult*. Philadelphia, PA: Lippincott Williams & Wilkins; 2011.

Doenges ME, Moorhouse MF, Murr AC. *Nursing Diagnosis Manual*. St Louis, MO: F.A. Davis; 2010.

Farmer DG, Anselmo DM, Ghobrial RM, et al. Liver transplantation for fulminant hepatic failure. *Ann Surg*. 2003;237:666-676.

Guyton AC, Hall JE. *Textboook of Medical Physiology*. 9th ed. Philadelphia, PA: W.B. Saunders Co; 1996.

Horne PM. Managing complications in patients with cirrhosis and hepatocellular cancer. *Am J Nurse Pract*. 2011;15:28-34.

Kelley WN. *Textbook of Internal Medicine*. 3rd ed. Philadelphia, PA: Lippincott-Raven; 1992.

McPhee SJ, Papadakis M, Rabow MW. *2011 Current Medical Diagnosis & Treatment*. New York: McGraw-Hill; 2011.

Phipps WJ, Monhahan FD, Sands JK, Marek JF, Neighbors M. *Medical-Surgical Nursing Health and Illness Perspectives*. 7th ed. St Louis, MO: Mosby; 2003.

Professional Guide to Signs and Symptoms. 5th ed. Philadelphia, PA: Lippincott Williams & Wilkins; 2009.

Sherman C. Staying up to date on managing hepatitis B. *Clin Advisor*. 2008;11:17-20.

Smith GD. Irritable bowel syndrome: quality of life and nursing interventions. *Br J Nurs*. 2006;15:1152-1156.

Taber's Cyclopedic Medical Dictionary. Philadelphia, PA: F.A. Davis; 2009.

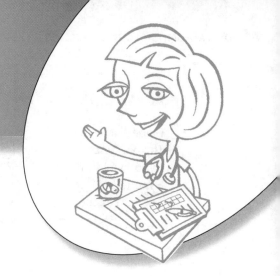

chapter 5

Endocrine System

LEARNING OBJECTIVES

At the end of this chapter, the reader/student will be able to:

- Analyze the functions of hormones secreted by the pituitary, thyroid, adrenal, and pancreas

- Describe the location of the endocrine glands and the physiologic functioning of each

- Discuss the common clinical manifestations and diagnostic tests used to identify endocrine dysfunction

- Compare the biological effects of excess and deficits of hormones in disease states

> ## KEY WORDS
>
> Diabetes Mellitus   Addison's Disease
> Thyroid Function   Cushing's Syndrome
> Hypothyroidism   Pancreas Function
> Hyperthyroidism   Pancreatitis
> Adrenal Function

Introduction

Endocrine pertains to a secretion of hormones into the bloodstream from a ductless gland. Together with the central nervous system (CNS), the endocrine system regulates the body's metabolic processes and maintains homeostasis. Endocrinopathy is any disease that results from a disorder of these glands. There may be hypersecretion or hyposecretion of the hormone, which will upset the homeostasis of the body and result in a disease state. The master gland is the hypothalamus, which is located in the midbrain and stimulates the anterior pituitary to produce various releasing and inhibitory hormones that affect glands and body processes. The hypothalamic-pituitary axis is important in the physiology of the endocrine system. This chapter will address diabetes mellitus, thyroid disorders, and adrenal disorders and pancreatitis.

Diabetes Mellitus

Diabetes mellitus (DM) involves dysfunction of the pancreas. The pancreas normally secretes insulin from the beta cells of the islet of Langerhans. After a meal when glucose levels are high in a nondiabetic person, the feedback system controls the glucose to rapidly return it to normal levels within 2 hours after a meal. The liver functions as a blood glucose buffer system. The glucose level rises after a big meal along with the rate of insulin secretion, and the increasing glucose is also absorbed in the gut and then stored as glycogen in the liver. Both insulin and glucagon function in a feedback mechanism to maintain normal blood glucose levels. Insulin ensures that the body is able to use glucose for energy. In DM there is diminished secretion of insulin, causing high glucose levels to persist as it is not absorbed, thereby decreasing the utilization of glucose by the body. Blood glucose levels can increase to 300–1200 mg/dL when normal levels are less than 105 mg/dL 2 hours after a meal. With no glucose in the body to burn for energy, the body burns fats and the increase in moving fats from fat storage results in abnormal fat metabolism and deposition of cholesterol in arterial walls. The body normally uses glucose for energy, but when the body depends on fat for energy the level of keto acids increases and ketoacidosis occurs. When glucose levels are high, the kidneys cannot keep up with reabsorbing the glucose from the glomerular filtrate. Glucose attracts water and osmotic diuresis occurs, resulting in polyuria (increased urination). DM can be caused by heredity (which plays a major role), viruses or the development of autoimmune antibodies, and obesity, which decreases the number of insulin receptors throughout the body.

Clinical Manifestations

High levels of glucose can result in dehydration of the tissue cells. As a result of these physiologic changes, the earliest symptoms experienced are polyuria (excessive urination), polydipsia (excessive thirst and drinking of water), polyphagia (excessive eating), loss of weight, and esthesia (lack of energy). By the time the disease becomes apparent, almost 80% of the beta cells are gone. Women may experience frequent yeast infections because of the high glucose level, which can be among the first indications that the person has DM. Patients who have DM can develop vision problems, neuropathy, kidney problems, and difficulty in healing sores.

Diagnostic Tests

DM is diagnosed by random and fasting blood glucose levels and symptoms experienced; glycosylated hemoglobin (HbA1c), which is utilized to determine glycemic control during the past 3 months (normal values are <6%, but in patients with poorly controlled diabetes it can be >12%); urinalysis; and lipid profile.

Treatment

Treatment is aimed at decreasing glucose levels using oral antiglycemic drugs such as sulfonylureas (Glucotrol, Diabinese) or other medications or through insulin replacement. Nutrition is important and the goal is to maintain an as nearly normal carbohydrate, fat, and protein metabolism as possible and to eat a well-balanced diabetic diet to prevent acute and chronic complications.

Nursing Interventions and Complications

Nurses assume a large portion of the responsibility for care and teaching and motivating diabetes patients to effectively manage their own disease, because it is a lifelong disorder. Nurses are knowledgeable about the signs and symptoms of hypoglycemia that can occur if too much insulin is given and the patient cannot eat, or when the patient has exercised a great deal, how there would be a decrease in the amount of insulin required. Nursing intervention is to give a short-acting carbohydrate such as milk or if severely low in the hospital setting a glucose tablet. Hyperglycemia can lead to a crisis and diabetic ketoacidosis and if not treated properly can lead to coma or death. This is caused when the insulin level is inadequate and high levels of glucose accumulate in the blood because glucose cannot be utilized by the cells in DM.

Nurses teach newly diagnosed diabetes patients how to use a glucometer (to measure glucose levels throughout the day); insulin administration; diabetic diet; side effects of hyperglycemia and hypoglycemic reactions and what to do when they experience symptoms; and about the potential complications on failure to follow close glycemic control (kidney disease, skin disease and delayed healing, cardiovascular disease, eye disease, and peripheral vascular disease). Further, nurses might refer patients to a podiatrist for foot care, to an ophthalmologist for eye care, and to a diabetic support group.

> ### CLINICAL ALERT
>
> *Late-stage complications of DM are pathologic changes in blood vessels including cranial, peripheral, and the lens of the eye, leading to hypertension, end-stage renal disease, blindness, peripheral neuropathy, amputations of lower extremities, myocardial infarction, and cerebrovascular accident. Nurses must work with DM patients to manage this disease by maintaining strict glycemic control and having frequent tests and follow-up to try to avoid these life-threatening consequences of DM.*

Thyroid Function

Approximately 93% of metabolically active hormone secreted by the thyroid gland is *thyroxine* whereas only 7% is *triiodothyronine*, commonly referred to as T3 and T4. To produce normal amounts of thyroxine, about

1 mg/wk of iodine is needed, and iodized table salt meets the requirement. Thyroid hormones maintain correct body metabolism by affecting carbohydrate metabolism, plasma and liver fats, basal metabolic rate, weight, cardiac output, CNS, sleep, and muscle function. The thyroid-stimulating hormone (TSH), also known as *thyrotropin*, is secreted by the anterior thyroid after stimulation by the hypothalamus, which releases thyroid-releasing hormone (TRH). This again reinforces the importance of the hypothalamic-pituitary axis. This is also on a feedback mechanism whereby increased thyroid hormone in the body fluids decreases the secretion of TSH. The feedback mechanism's effect is to maintain a constant concentration of free thyroid hormones in the body fluids. The thyroid gland is located at the center of the base of the neck.

Hypothyroidism

Hypothyroidism may be the result of an autoimmune disease against the thyroid gland, which destroys it and causes diminished or absent secretion of hormone thyroid. Low concentrations of thyroid hormones increase the plasma concentration of cholesterol, phospholipids, and triglycerides; the metabolic rate decreases, leading to increased body weight, sluggish muscles, and sleepiness and makes the patient feel cold. This can be caused by primary hypothyroidism (decreased thyroid hormone levels) or by hypothalamic-pituitary dysfunction or secondary hypothyroidism.

The hypometabolic state is caused by a deficiency of thyroid hormones. Hashimoto thyroiditis accounts for most cases of hypothyroidism in the United States and is an autoimmune inflammatory disorder that may or may not result in a goiter (enlargement of the gland) or thyroid nodules. The etiology is uncertain and may have a genetic component (Figure 5–1).

Clinical Manifestations

Myxedema can develop insidiously with slowing down of physical and mental activity and is associated with symptoms of periorbital edema; fatigue; coarse, dry skin; weight gain; cold intolerance; coarse hair, skin, and facial features; hair loss; hand pain and paresthesias (carpal tunnel syndrome); increased weakness, lethargy, cold intolerance; decreased memory; and constipation and can also have swelling of hands and feet. In women, menstrual irregularities might be present.

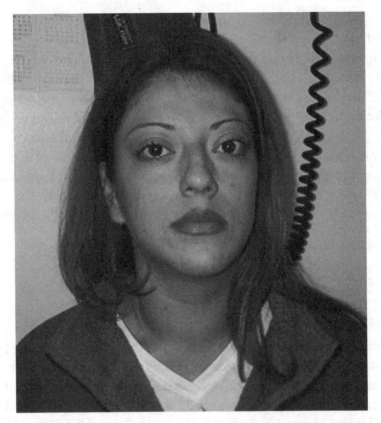

FIGURE 5-1 • This patient displays the following common findings of Graves' disease (GD): Lid retraction and mild proptosis (exophthalmus), particularly evident on the left eye, and goiter. (Reproduced with permission from Usatine RP, et al. *The Color Atlas of Family Medicine.* New York: McGraw-Hill; 2009, figure 217-1. Courtesy of Dan Stulberg, MD.)

Diagnostic Tests

Diagnosis is made by elevated serum levels of TSH and low levels of T4 and T3. Measurement of TSH levels is usually the first test, as the level rises as soon as the circulating levels of thyroid hormones are low. Lipid profile testing may also reveal an increase in low-density lipoprotein (LDL) and decrease in high-density lipoprotein (HDL) cholesterol and liver enzymes, and the person may have hyponatremia, hypoglycemia, and anemia. CT or MRI can be taken if the patient has a goiter.

Treatment

Treatment is aimed at replacing thyroid hormone T4 with levothyroxine using medications such as Levoxyl, Synthroid, or Levothroid.

Nursing Implications and Complications

Nurses must assess patients for constipation due to decreased gastrointestinal motility, depression, weight gain, fatigue, and other signs. Nurses must especially be alert to myxedema coma, which is a medical emergency that can lead to death and where stresses such as infection or exposure to cold may lead to prolonged, severe symptoms of hypothyroidism with depressed respiration rates and decreased cardiac output. Nurses teach patients the importance of continued hormone replacement therapy. Nurses should be skilled at assessing the thyroid and identifying patients with goiters and should be able to assess whether the goiter interferes with breathing or swallowing.

> ### CLINICAL ALERT
>
> *Patients with severe hypothyroidism have an increased risk of bacterial pneumonia and megacolon. Untreated or inadequate dosing during pregnancy can cause miscarriage. Myxedema crisis is life-threatening hypothyroidism and patients can have confusion to coma and have hypoglycemia, hypothermia, and hypoventilation, which can require mechanical ventilation. Nurses must not give opioids to patients with myxedema because even an average dose can result in death.*

Hyperthyroidism

Hyperthyroidism (also called thyrotoxicosis) occurs when an excess of circulating thyroid hormones is produced. It is relatively common and much more likely found in women than men. There is an increased production of TSH. Thyroid hormone enhances sensitivity of catecholamines, and an excessive amount of the hormone leads to a hypermetabolic state with heat intolerance, nervousness, tremor, increased appetite, weight loss, excessive sweating, stare, muscle weakness, tachycardia, dyspnea on exertion, emotional lability, and possible frequent bowel movements. Graves disease is an autoimmune disorder and is the most common disorder causing hyperthyroidism and accounts for about 90% of cases in people younger than age 40 years. Graves disease clinically exhibits diffuse thyroid enlargement (smooth diffuse goiter), ophthalmopathy (bulging eyes), and occasionally pretibial myxedema (reddened, mildly scaly plaques on the skin from the ankles to the pretibial area). The first sign is a suppressed TSH level. Hyperthyroidism causes increased activity of the sympathetic nervous system and affects fat and carbohydrate metabolism.

There is a shortened systolic interval, increasing cardiac output, which may lead to congestive heart failure. Excess thyroid hormone can increase the mobilization of calcium from the bone, and the increased urinary excretion of calcium and phosphorus may decrease bone mass.

Clinical Manifestations

Nervousness, increased sweating, heat intolerance, palpitations, tachycardia, fatigue, weakness, weight loss, tremor, emotional lability, increased appetite, and warm moist skin are generally seen, with some patients having exophthalmos and goiter.

Diagnostic Tests

Hyperthyroidism or thyrotoxicosis is diagnosed by elevated serum levels of T4 and T3 and suppressed (<0.1 µU/mL) levels of TSH, serum antithyroid antibodies, thyroid sonogram, or radioisotope scanning to identify thyroid growth. There may also be elevated levels of alkaline phosphatase and angiotensin-converting enzyme that may persist even after treatment, although the pathophysiologic reasons for these two signs remain unclear.

Treatment

Treatment involves antithyroid medications such as propylthiouracil (PTU); methimazole (Tapazole); propranolol, which may be given for symptomatic relief until hyperthyroidism is under control; radioactive iodine therapy, which may destroy cells to reduce the thyroid hormone production (not to be done in pregnancy); and surgical removal of part of the thyroid, if patient is younger than age 40 years and has repeated relapses. For acute progressive exophthalmos, intravenous methylprednisone is given.

Nursing Interventions and Complications

Hyperthyroidism is a hypermetabolic disease. If hyperthyroidism is untreated or is unrecognized, it can lead to a thyroid storm, which is an acute exacerbation of symptoms that can result in death. Precipitating factors leading to thyroid storm can be brought on by a stressful event such as surgery, trauma, or infection. (An example could be a diabetes patient with ketoacidosis.) Patients with any thyroid condition should be taught about which symptoms would require seeing their endocrinologists and for which they need to seek emergency care.

Reinforce the need to take their daily prescribed thyroid medications. Educate patients about supportive treatments such as nutrients and vitamins, especially for those with hyperactive thyroid disease, and about what the lab tests are for. Teach patients that certain medications may result in possible interactions, and thyroid values should be closely monitored when taking such medication as oral anticoagulants, oral hypoglycemic agents, estrogen; oral contraceptives and iron may decrease absorption if taken at the same time.

> ## CLINICAL ALERT
>
> *Complications include cardiac arrhythmias and heart failure, thyroid crisis, ophthalmopathy (disease of the eye), and paralysis along with hypokalemia. Despite treatment for long-term hyperthyroidism, women experience an increased long-term risk of death such as cardiac arrhythmia and stroke. Nurses need to closely monitor patients with hyperthyroidism and treat with appropriate medications.*

Adrenal Function

There are two adrenal glands located above the kidneys. The outer part of the gland is the cortex, comprising about 80% of the gland, and it secretes steroid hormones: the mineralocorticoids (aldosterone), androgens, and glucocorticoids (cortisol). The medulla makes up the rest of the gland and secretes epinephrine, norepinephrine, and dopamine. Aldosterone regulates the absorption of sodium and the excretion of potassium by the kidneys. The androgens produced are in small amounts and play a minor role in maintaining secondary sex characteristics, and a small amount of estrogen is converted peripherally from the androgens (androstenedione), which becomes the major source of estrogen in the postmenopausal woman. The weak androgens are converted in peripheral tissue to stronger ones such as testosterone, which causes an androgenic effect. The glucocorticoids have an antiinflammatory and growth-suppressing effect. They also increase blood glucose levels by the process of gluconeogenesis (formation of glucose from excess amino acids and fats), which occurs in the liver and stimulates the breakdown of increased protein and mobilizes free fatty acids and increased cholesterol. Cortisol is necessary for maintenance of life and protection from stress and helps to maintain blood pressure and heart function. The adrenal cortex is controlled by the secretion of adrenocorticotropic hormone (ACTH) from the anterior pituitary gland.

The medulla secretes the catecholamines epinephrine (adrenaline) and norepi-nephrine, which is controlled by the sympathetic nervous system. Epinephrine is about 75%–85% of the catecholamine secreted and is secreted in the body's response to the emotional stress of a fight-or-flight response. It causes dilation of the bronchioles, increased blood pressure and heart rate, and increased blood glucose level. The norepinephrine causes tachycardia, vasoconstriction, and tachypnea. Dopamine is a catecholamine that influences the emotional state.

Addison's Disease

Addison's disease is the failure of the adrenal cortices to produce adrenocorti-cal hormones and this in turn most likely causes atrophy of the adrenal cortices. Autoimmune destruction of the adrenals is the most common cause of Addison disease. With the lack of aldosterone, there is a greatly decreased renal tubular sodium reabsorption, which allows sodium and chloride ions and water to be lost into the urine, causing decreased extracellular fluid volume. Hyponatre-mia, hyperkalemia, and mild acidosis occur because of failure of potassium to be excreted in exchange for sodium reabsorption. The loss of cortisol results in failure to maintain normal blood glucose by gluconeogenesis and it reduces the mobilization of proteins and fats from the tissue. There is sluggishness due to lack of energy and weakness in muscles. It also makes the person with Addison's highly susceptible to times of stress, whereby even a mild respiratory infection may result in death. There is also increased melanin production in mucous membranes and the skin. This might happen because the feedback mechanism to the pituitary is not working and there is an overproduction of ACTH, which may stimulate the production of MSH (melanocyte-stimulating hormone), which produces melanin under the skin and discoloration or blotchiness. If a person remains untreated, Addison disease can result in death.

Clinical Manifestations

Weakness, fatigue, weight loss, increased pigmentation (especially increases in pressure areas and nipples), anorexia, nausea, vomiting, decreased cold toler-ance, salt craving, and hair loss in females are common.

Diagnostic Tests

Low serum sodium, elevated potassium level, metabolic acidosis, elevated blood urea nitrogen (BUN) and calcium, low cortisol levels, and elevated

ACTH levels can confirm diagnosis. Complete blood count (CBC; because white blood cell count is elevated) and glucose level must be examined.

Treatment

The treatment involves replacing cortisol and aldosterone for life. Hypofunctioning of the adrenal medulla, which secretes epinephrine and norepinephrine, does not seem to produce any known physiologic problems.

Nursing Implications and Complications

Nursing diagnosis is based on history, and deficit in fluid volume should be treated by encouraging fluid intake and monitoring fluid status frequently. Nurses also assess a patient's knowledge of the disease and explain symptoms and the need to continue glucocorticoids and mineral corticoids every day for life. The patient should be advised to reduce stress and conserve energy.

CLINICAL ALERT

Adrenal crisis (Addisonian crisis) is a potential life-threatening critical care issue and often occurs in undiagnosed Addison disease or those who stop taking their medication, or during stress such as trauma or surgery. Management includes prompt rehydration, administration of stress doses of intravenous hydrocortisone, correction of electrolyte levels, and intravenous glucose if the patient is hypoglycemic.

Cushing's Syndrome

Cushing's syndrome is caused by hypersecretion of the adrenal cortex and may result from a cortisol-secreting tumor or hyperplasia of both adrenal cortices. This in turn causes increased production of ACTH. There is mobilization of fat in the lower body, with additional deposits in the thoracic and upper abdomen region. The extra hormonal secretion results in an edematous or fat appearance of the face. The androgenic potency of some of the hormones can lead to acne and hirsutism (excessive hair growth in the face and in other areas of the body, especially in women). The abundance of cortisol can greatly increase blood glucose levels, and after meals even more so. The increased glucocorticoid levels cause protein catabolism (breaking down), which results in decreased tissue protein almost everywhere in the body, causing muscle weakness and a weakened immune system, which can lead to death due to infection. Cushing's

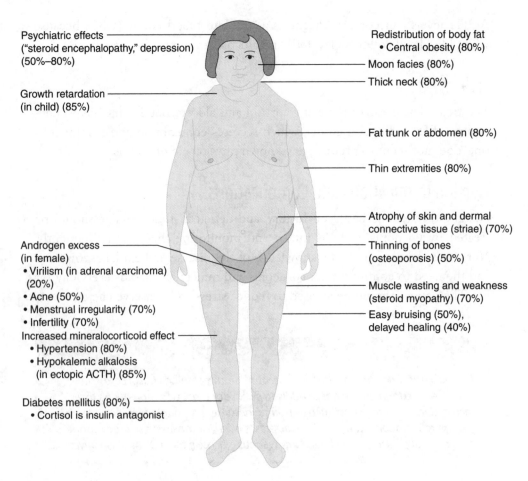

Psychiatric effects ("steroid encephalopathy," depression) (50%–80%)

Growth retardation (in child) (85%)

Androgen excess (in female)
• Virilism (in adrenal carcinoma) (20%)
• Acne (50%)
• Menstrual irregularity (70%)
• Infertility (70%)
Increased mineralocorticoid effect
• Hypertension (80%)
• Hypokalemic alkalosis (in ectopic ACTH) (85%)

Diabetes mellitus (80%)
• Cortisol is insulin antagonist

Redistribution of body fat
• Central obesity (80%)
Moon facies (80%)
Thick neck (80%)

Fat trunk or abdomen (80%)

Thin extremities (80%)

Atrophy of skin and dermal connective tissue (striae) (70%)
Thinning of bones (osteoporosis) (50%)

Muscle wasting and weakness (steroid myopathy) (70%)
Easy bruising (50%), delayed healing (40%)

FIGURE 5–2 • Typical findings in Cushing's syndrome. (Reproduced with permission from McPhee SJ, Hammer GD, eds. *Pathophysiology of Disease: An Introduction to Clinical Medicine.* 6th ed. New York: McGraw-Hill; 2009, figure 21-11.)

syndrome can develop in different ways: ACTH overproduction; ectopic ACTH overproduction by tumors; independent cortisol-secreting adrenal, or very rarely an ovarian tumor. A high cortisol level is used to diagnose Cushing's but then the etiology must be determined, which is done by the dexamethasone suppression test and the basal-state blood ACTH level. Most people with Cushing's syndrome have a pituitary microadenoma that results in a loss of the feedback mechanism to control ACTH secretion (Figure 5–2).

Clinical Manifestations

Moon face (facial fat), increased adipose tissue in the neck (buffalo hump) and trunk, acne, weight gain, hypertension, osteoporosis, striae on the skin (purple lines on areas such as abdomen, breasts, legs), diabetes or glucose intolerance, hirsutism, easy bruising of the skin, lability of mood, and menstrual disorders are the main clinical manifestations.

Diagnostic Tests

Twenty-four-hour 17-hydroxycorticosteroids and cortisol test, plasma cortisol, plasma ACTH concentration, hyperglycemia, hyperlipidemia, and 2-day dexamethasone suppression tests can ascertain a diagnosis of Cushing's syndrome.

Treatment

Treatment is often surgical, and generally microsurgery through the transsphenoidal pituitary is utilized and cures about 80% of patients with Cushing's syndrome. Radiation may also be used as a treatment. Medical use of adrenocortical inhibitors has not been too successful. Hirsutism is treated by laser hair removal or waxing, and some shave the excess hair growth. Of course, if diabetes or hypertension develops, it must be treated.

Nursing Interventions and Complications

Nurses working with patients with Cushing's syndrome should be aware of the complications associated with this disease and teach the patient about the disease. The complications are osteoporosis and pathologic fractures caused by increased calcium reabsorption from bone, which may require patients to take supplements or bisphosphonates (Actonel, Fosamax, Boniva), peptic ulcer caused by increased gastric secretions, and impaired glucose tolerance. Nurses are responsible for health promotions in these patients. Those with Cushing's syndrome may have frequent infections and slow wound healing and hypertension because of sodium and water retention, which may also lead to heart disease. During an acute period of illness, the primary focus of the nurse should be to support coping and help the patient deal with body image changes, restore fluid balance, and prevent infections or injury.

CLINICAL ALERT

Cushing's syndrome, if untreated, produces serious morbidity and even death. A patient may suffer from complications of hypertension or diabetes. Nurses must know the signs and symptoms, screening tests, and treatment of patients with Cushing's syndrome and assess for signs of complications.

Pancreas Function

The pancreas is both an exocrine and endocrine gland and the master digestive gland of the body. As an exocrine gland, it secretes digestive enzymes necessary for the breakdown of protein, starch, fat, and fat-soluble vitamins. The enzymes secreted are amylase, which breaks down carbohydrate; trypsin, which breaks down protein; and lipase, which breaks down fat. The pancreas is rich in arterial blood from the branches of the celiac and mesenteric arteries. As an endocrine gland, the small clusters of cells called islets of Langerhans are composed of alpha cells, which secrete glucagon, and beta cells, which secrete insulin when glucose levels rise. As discussed in the section on DM, it is the dysfunction of the endocrine portion of the pancreas that results in diabetes.

Pancreatitis

Pancreatitis is an inflammatory process arising in the pancreas. It can range in severity from a mild self-limiting disease to severe disease with potentially severe complications. Gallstone disease and excessive alcohol use account for 70%–80% of cases of pancreatitis. People with genetic hyperlipidemia with very high triglyceride levels can also develop pancreatitis. Several drugs have been implicated as causes of pancreatitis, such as sulfonamides, methyldopa, metronidazole, erythromycin, and acetaminophen. Pancreatitis can be acute and may be interstitial, causing fluid accumulation and swelling due to release of digestive enzymes, or necrotizing, causing death and tissue damage. If there is damage to the islets of Langerhans, DM may develop. Chronic pancreatitis is characterized by bouts of mild to severe epigastric pain and often occurs in alcoholics after years of drinking, which results in calcification or fibrosis of the pancreas. Gallbladder disease can cause pancreatitis when a gallstone blocks the main secretory duct from the pancreas as well as the common bile duct, causing the pancreatic enzymes to be blocked. This blockage of enzymes in the pancreas can digest and destroy portions of the pancreas. Often surgical removal of the gallbladder stone or stones must be performed. The role of alcohol in pancreatitis is that it is toxic and can stimulate pancreatic enzymes and cause spasms. The large release of the enzymes before they reach the duodenum is a major component of this disease. There are more women with biliary tract pancreatitis and more men with alcohol-related pancreatitis.

Clinical Manifestations

In pancreatitis, there is a steady, severe epigastric pain radiating to the back that is worse when lying supine, nausea and vomiting, hypokalemia, mild abdominal distention, diminished bowel sounds, fever (100°–101°F), pain worsened by eating or by drinking alcohol, and abdominal tenderness on palpation.

Diagnostic Tests

Serum amylase, lipase (will be elevated), elevated alanine aminotransferase (ALT) and aspartate aminotransferase (AST), glucose, x-ray, ultrasonography or CT scan, and endoscopic retrograde cholangiopancreatography (ERCP) are the tests performed for making a diagnosis.

Treatment

Mild disease is treated with rest, maintaining the patient on a nothing-by-mouth diet, and pain medication. In severe disease such as necrotizing pancreatitis, leakage of fluids may occur, and large amounts of intravenous fluids are given and the patient is monitored in the intensive care unit. Exploratory surgery may be necessary in cases of gallbladder stones.

Nursing Interventions and Complications

Controlling pain is a priority in these patients, in addition to monitoring and maintaining fluid and electrolyte balance. Usually patients are given nothing by mouth, so maintaining adequate nutrition by nasogastric tube or intravenous fluids is very important. Nurses should educate the patients about pancreatitis and the planned diagnostic tests or surgical intervention, address the unhealthy lifestyle in the alcoholic and refer for treatment or counseling. Further, it is important to assess lab values and continually assess patients' vital signs, perform palpation of abdomen to check for increased rigidity, and assess for third spacing, falling urine output, or increased abdominal girth and increased pain. About 25% of patients who experience acute pancreatitis develop complications and in this group death may result; therefore, careful close assessment by nurses is paramount. If surgery is indicated, pre- and postoperative teaching and care is important.

CLINICAL ALERT

Necrotic pancreatitis may require surgery to remove the necrotic area. Patients requiring surgery for fulminant disease are acutely ill with hypovolemic shock, oliguria, ascites, jaundice, and respiratory failure. Nurses must manage the postoperative patient and be acutely aware of the complications that can develop with pancreatitis.

CASE STUDY

LP is a patient who is complaining of chronic fatigue, increased thirst, frequent urination, and constant hunger. She also mentions that she has frequent yeast infections. She recently started smoking again because of stress related to family matters. She also started working and is having difficulty reading numbers and making mistakes at work. She is too tired to exercise after work and family responsibilities and also complains that her feet hurt and often "burn or feel like pins are in them." Her diet is high in carbohydrates. When you assess her history, you find that she has gained considerable weight since her last child and is 5'2" and weighs 172 lbs. Her B/P (blood pressure) is 154/98 mm Hg. She also states she always feels cold and that she is experiencing some hair loss. When you look at her lab values, her fasting plasma glucose is 188 mg/dL, HbA1c is 10.4; her urinalysis shows a high glucose level, cholesterol level is 260 mg/dL, triglycerides 366 mg/dL, LDL 155 mg/dL, HDL 34 mg/dL, and TSH 11.4 IU/L.

QUESTIONS

1. Identify the signs and symptoms used to diagnosis DM.
2. Which of the symptoms that LP reports suggest that she has some form of neuropathy?
3. What are some other symptoms related to DM?
4. What are the 3 behaviors that you would speak to the patient about regarding health promotion?
5. What comorbid disease may she also have?

Suggested Readings

Bartol T. Motivating patients to behavior change: tools and techniques for patients with diabetes. *American Journal for Nurse Practitioners*. 2011;15(5/6):14-23.

Burch WM. *Endocrinology for the House Officer*. 2nd ed. Baltimore, MD: Williams & Wilkins; 1988.

Corall AH, Mulby AG. *Primary Care Medicine*. 4th ed. Philadelphia, PA: Lippincott Williams & Wilkins; 2000.

Crutchlow EM, Dudnac PJ, MacAvoy S, Madara BR. *Quick Look: Nursing Pathophysiology*. Thorofare, NJ: Slack Inc; 2002.

Dambro MR. *Griffith's 5 Minute Clinical Consult*. Baltimore, MD: Williams & Wilkins; 2011.

Dancer S, Courtney M. Improving diabetes patient outcomes: framing research into chronic care model. *J Am Acad Nurse Pract*. 2010;22(11):580-585.

Dillon RM. *Nursing Health Assessment: A Critical Thinking Case Studies Approach*. 2nd ed. Philadelphia, PA: F.A. Davis; 2007.

Guyton AC, Hall JE. *Textbook of Medical Physiology*. 9th ed. Philadelphia, PA: W.B. Saunders; 1996.

Irland NB. The story of type 2 diabetes. *Nurs Women's Health*. 2011;15(2):153-165.

Kelley WN. *Textbook of Internal Medicine*. 3rd ed. Philadelphia, PA: Lippincott-Raven; 1992.

Pathophysiology Made Incredibly Easy. 4th ed. Philadelphia, PA: Wolters Kluwer/ Lippincott Williams & Wilkins; 2009.

Phipps WJ, Monhahan FD, Sands JK, Marek JF, Neighbors M. *Medical-Surgical Nursing Health and Illness Perspectives*. 7th ed. St. Louis, MO: Mosby; 2003.

Professional Guide to Signs and Symptoms. 5th ed. Philadelphia, PA: Lippincott Williams & Wilkins; 2009.

Taber's Cyclopedic Medical Dictionary. Philadelphia, PA: F.A. Davis; 2009.

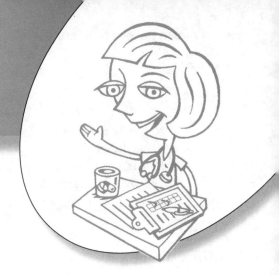

chapter **6**

Genitourinary System

LEARNING OBJECTIVES

At the end of this chapter, the reader/student will be able to:

- Describe the physiology of the upper and lower urinary tract, including the bladder and kidney
- Identify urinary tract problems and treatments
- Correlate diagnostic tests for urinary tract disorders
- List the types of renal dialysis

KEY WORDS

Nephrotic Syndrome
Renal Dialysis
Renal Calculi
Urinary Tract Infections

Interstitial Cystitis
Glomerulonephritis
Renal Failure

Introduction

The urinary system is composed of two kidneys, two ureters, which comprise the upper urinary tract, and a bladder and urethra, which comprise the lower urinary tract. The kidneys are the most important part of the urinary system. One function is to rid the body of waste materials that are either ingested or produced through metabolism, which is accomplished by filtering plasma and removing substances from the filtrate at different rates, depending on what the body needs. Another function that is especially critical is to control the volume and composition of the body fluids. All water and electrolytes in the body are balanced between input and output by the kidneys. The kidneys serve multiple functions such as the regulation of water and electrolyte balance; regulation of body fluid osmolarity and electrolyte concentrations; regulation of acid-base balance; regulation of arterial pressure; secretion of hormones; and gluconeogenesis (formation of glucose from excess amino acids, fats, and other noncarbohydrate sources). The kidneys have three distinct areas: the renal cortex, where most of the nephrons (the functioning units of the kidney, and each kidney contains about 1 million nephrons) are located; the renal medulla, which consists of triangular wedges that are segments of nephrons and collecting ducts, and the renal sinus, which is a cavity filled with blood. The kidneys are highly vascular organs. The nephrons decrease in number as one ages and cannot be regenerated if lost. Each nephron has two components: (1) glomerulus (glomerular capillaries), through which the large amount of fluid is filtered from the blood, and (2) a long tubule in which the filtered fluid is converted into urine. The glomerular capillaries, like most capillaries, are relatively impermeable to proteins, so the glomerular filtrate is essentially protein-free and devoid of cellular elements, including red blood cells. The glomerular filtration rate (GFR) is determined by the balance of hydrostatic and colloid osmotic forces acting across the capillary membrane. The ability of the kidneys to conserve water and electrolytes is important for survival. The proximal convoluted tubule reabsorbs most of the water, up to 80% of filtered sodium and most of filtered potassium, bicarbonate, chloride, phosphate, glucose, and amino acids. Another mechanism that prevents water and electrolyte depletion is a hormone produced in the hypothalamus that regulates salt and water balance called antidiuretic hormone (ADH) or vasopressin. ADH is released if water intake is too low or water loss is high in order to make the kidneys conserve water. To maintain normal pH, which is 7.35–7.45, the bicarbonate-to-carbon dioxide ratio must be at 20:1, and the respiratory system and the kidneys work together. The lungs add carbon dioxide to the blood and the kidneys either secrete or retain bicarbonate and hydrogen ions in response to Ph of the blood.

The kidneys also regulate calcium and phosphorus reciprocally. Aldosterone is a hormone produced in the adrenal cortex. The major stimulus for aldosterone production is a reflex by the kidney. Cells in the kidney monitor sodium levels and blood volume. When either of these decrease, the cells in the kidney secrete a protein called rennin. Renin acts on the angiotensinogen, a plasma formed in the liver to produce angiotensin I, but when it is not sufficient for vasoconstriction amino acids split to form angiotensin II. Angiotensin II is a powerful renal vasoconstrictor which is formed in the kidneys as well as the systemic circulation. Increases in this hormone will raise the glomerular hydrostatic pressure while reducing renal blood flow. The regulation of angiotensin II is stimulated in response to volume depletion or low sodium and will raise the glomerular hydrostatic pressure while reducing renal blood flow. The regulation of angiotensin II is stimulated in response to volume depletion or low sodium diets, when an increase in the hormone will help preserve the GFR, and will maintain normal excretion of metabolic waste products, such as urea and creatinine. Angiotensin II through constriction of the efferent arterioles causes an increased resorption of sodium and water, which helps to maintain blood volume and blood pressure. The kidneys are crucial for red cell production when decreased tissue oxygenation occurs. The kidneys respond by producing about 90% of the body's erythropoietin, which stimulates the bone marrow to produce erythrocytes. When the kidneys fail and anemia results, treatment of a genetically engineered erythropoietin (Epogen or Procrit) is given.

Urine from the kidneys propels through the ureters by peristaltic action and is collected in the bladder, which stores the urine. The urge to urinate usually occurs when the bladder has about 300 mL of urine. It is important to understand the physiologic function of the kidneys and urinary system to fully understand the states of pathology.

Nephrotic Syndrome

This is caused by damage to the capillary membrane which maintains the balance of hydrostatic and colloid (protein) osmotic pressure. The damage results in excessive permeability, which permits proteins through and proteinuria occurs. Depending on the degree of damage to the membrane, there may be only low-molecular-weight proteins such as albumin and transferrin, but with severe damage there may be high-molecular-weight proteins as well as albumin passing through the damaged membrane. These patients also have sodium and water retention, hyperlipidemia, lipiduria, vulnerability to infection, and thrombolytic complications due to low albumin and loss of antithrombin. Edema results from the renal salt retention and the decreased osmotic pressure. This can be caused by primary renal disease or from other diseases such as diabetic nephropathy, lupus nephropathy, infection, cancer, preeclampsia, as well as drug addiction or nephrotoxic drugs.

The amount of protein that can be lost in the urine can be as much as 40 g a day. Immunologic studies have also shown in some cases, abnormal immune reactions have resulted from antibody attack on the membrane.

Clinical Manifestations

Abdominal distention; abdominal fluid shift; generalized edema (anasarca); puffy eyelids; scrotal swelling; weight gain; shortness of breath; pulmonary edema hypertension; normal or greatly altered urine volume; loss of appetite; fatigue; and protein in the urine (a sign of infection due to the loss of immunoglobulins, which are plasma proteins) are generally observed.

Diagnostic Tests

To confirm diagnosis, the following tests are undertaken: urinalysis, blood chemistries for albumin (to determine loss), lipids (as protein is lost, hyperlipidemia occurs), renal biopsy, blood count and coagulation screen, renal function tests: blood urea nitrogen (BUN), creatinine, blood glucose to rule out diabetes, renal ultrasound, chest x-ray to rule out pleural effusion or infection, and Doppler or magnetic resonance imaging (MRI) if a thrombosis is suspected.

Treatment

Treatment first line is salt restriction, and diuretics and statins (which have been shown to improve endothelial function and decrease proteinuria), and angiotensin-converting enzyme (ACE) inhibitors (e.g., Lotensin, Vasotec, Altace), or angiotensin II receptor blocker (ARB) inhibitors (e.g., Diovan, Avapro, Benicar), and corticosteroids. Replace the protein lost in urine to avoid a negative nitrogen balance. In patients with serum albumin levels of <2 g/dL, which can make the patient hypercoagulable, anticoagulant therapy is used for evidence of thrombus.

Nursing Interventions and Complications

Maintain the patient on a low-sodium diet and often high-protein diets are also ordered. Weigh the patient every day to ensure adequate nutrition and weight gain from intake greater than output, maintain intact skin especially because of edema, explain tests the patient may undergo, as well as explain all medications and what they are treating. Monitor the patient for infection and especially when on corticosteroids that can mask an infection, monitor lab results and urine for protein loss, maintain strict intake and output records, and assess respiratory status and blood pressure. The nurse needs to explain to the patient that the effect of nephrotic syndrome may result in the need for dialysis, and this complication may also require a renal transplant.

> ### CLINICAL ALERT
>
> *Nephrotic syndrome may lead to kidney failure and complications of fluid overload due to the protein shifts. The patient may also become hypovolemic. These patients will require dialysis and eventual kidney transplant. Nurses closely monitor patients with nephrotic syndrome and replace fluids and protein and monitor kidney function. Nurses also manage patients undergoing dialysis.*

Renal Dialysis

Renal dialysis is also called renal substitution therapy as it is used to improve the abnormalities that accompany renal failure. However, all available forms of dialysis provide only crude salt, water, and toxin removal. When compared with normal kidneys, clearance of most substances, including medications and metabolic by-products, is much less efficient and some degree of plasma toxins persist even with the best of regimes. Two major methods for accomplishing dialysis is hemodialysis and peritoneal dialysis, which are both effective in acute and chronic renal failure. **Hemodialysis** is an extracorporeal therapy in which blood is removed from the body and diffused across a semipermeable membrane to modify the chemical composition of the blood and then the blood is returned in a continuous manner over a 2- to 4-hour period. The continuous flow of 200 to 450 mL of blood per minute through an extracorporeal circuit is technically demanding and requires close monitoring by the mechanical sensors as well as by registered nurses (RNs) skilled and specially trained in dialysis. Hemodialysis is dependent on a reliable access to the bloodstream. Short-term access can be achieved by a specialized dual-lumen catheter placed temporarily in a high-flow central vein. A more permanent access for long-term dialysis is achieved surgically by creating a fistula between a peripheral artery and a vein; typically, the radial artery and cephalic vein are used.

Continuous renal replacement therapy (CRRT) provides 8–24 hours of continuous ultrafiltration of plasma, which pass through a hemofilter—a semipermeable membrane that clears uremic toxins. The ultrafiltration system is composed of outflow and return tubing. Arterial and venous access is needed. Blood is removed from the body and its volume is altered by the ultrafiltration of the plasma water across the semipermeable membrane where electrolytes, water, and other solutes are removed. The volume removed is replaced by a synthetic electrolyte solution that is similar to plasma in electrolytes and water with no protein. The clearance of the toxins, therefore, is equal to the amount of plasma water removed per unit of time because the plasma water is replaced by an equal volume of fluid that does not contain the toxins. Hemofiltration can be divided into two categories: continuous arteriovenous hemofiltration (CAVH) and continuous venovenous filtration (CVVH). Removal of plasma water and electrolytes is a gradual process that closely resembles the process in the kidney, so there are no rapid fluctuations in fluid and electrolytes as it occurs by diffusion and convection, which is the force through the fibers and is dependent on the blood pressure creating hydrostatic pressure within the hemofilter. CRRT is recommended for patients with advanced renal failure who are too unstable to undergo hemodialysis or peritoneal dialysis. Others who could benefit from CRRT are those patients with abdominal wounds, cerebral edema, or those with severe cardiac disease. The ultrafiltration system consists of an arterial access tube, a venous access tube connected by the filter, and an access for the ultrafiltrate with a bag to collect the toxins and material to be discarded. There is also a tube for heparin.

Peritoneal dialysis involves the placement of an aqueous solution dialysate into the peritoneal cavity, where it bathes the capillaries on the visceral mesenteric and parietal surfaces. The capillary walls and elements of the peritoneal surface act as a semipermeable membrane, across which solutes and water move by diffusion. It is used to treat acute and chronic renal failure. This can be done continuously, usually up to 36 hours or intermittently. A small incision is made in the abdomen below the umbilicus and a multilumen catheter is inserted into the peritoneal cavity. Warmed sterile dialysate (fluid used to remove the toxins) is attached by the tubing and is run in rapidly. The tubing is then clamped, allowing osmosis and diffusion of particles, for approximately 20–30 minutes and then the tube is unclamped to allow the fluid to drain by gravity from the peritoneal cavity. This process is repeated several times. There are benefits to peritoneal dialysis, and patients can learn continuous cyclic treatments for home self-dialysis. The other benefits are as follows: there are steady blood chemistry findings; patients can be taught and it can be done anywhere as there is no need for a dialysis machine; and there are less dietary restrictions because there is loss of protein in the dialysate and so a high-protein diet is permitted.

In the emergency setting, the choice of renal substitution therapy must meet the immediate medical needs of the patient and pose the least risk for complication.

Clinical Manifestations

Kidney failure requiring dialysis presents by symptoms of elevation of BUN due to decreased GFR, hyperkalemia, and loss of sodium (in late-stage renal failure, the excretion of sodium and water becomes limited and restriction of sodium and water become necessary; anemia, fatigue, itching from increased toxins; shortness of breath and cardiomyopathy due to fluid overload; metabolic acidosis due to the kidneys' inability to excrete ammonia, and loss of the bicarbonate (patient can have a smell of ammonia); uric acid level rises as urate excretion fails; edema; hiccups and nausea; muscle cramps and tetany due to hypocalcemia; confusion.

Diagnostic Tests

Symptoms of oliguria or changes in urinary function as well as the symptoms described in the Clinical Manifestations section should be noted. Calculate the GFR, assess urine for white and red blood cells (WBC/RBC), and electrolytes (sodium, creatinine, urea); do a 24-hour urinalysis for protein and creatinine; blood test for anemia and bleeding time; blood tests for BUN, creatinine, potassium level, calcium level, phosphate, and metabolic acidosis; computed tomographic (CT) scan to assess for cysts, neoplasm, or renal artery stenosis; renal biopsy; and intravenous pyelography (IVP).

Treatment

Renal failure dialysis is employed to act as the kidneys to remove waste products and excess electrolytes in the blood. Other indications are uremic symptoms such as pericarditis, encephalopathy or coagulopathy, fluid overload, and severe metabolic acidosis. In end-stage renal disease, kidney transplant is the only chance of cure and of increasing life expectancy. Only 50% of end-stage renal disease patients are candidates for renal transplantation.

Nursing Implications and Complications

Nurses monitor fluid status by assessing edema and monitoring intake and output as well as monitoring the patient for adequate nutrition, changes in mental functioning, blood pressure, cardiac status, smell on breath of ammonia, weight, ecchymosis, weakness and muscle tremors, and any signs of infection. Monitor laboratory results for BUN, potassium, complete blood count (CBC), creatinine and sodium levels, and pH level. Help the patient and family to cope with the symptoms of the illness that may alter the person's mental status and personality and also encourage the patient to continue activities of daily living (ADLs), and walking should be encouraged. Nurses also perform dialysis and teach patients what signs to look for that indicates it is time for their dialysis. Nurses closely monitor the patient during dialysis, maintain the hemodialysis machines because if any disinfectant is left in the machine and the next patient gets an accidental disinfectant infusion, it can result in metabolic complications, pulmonary symptoms, and even death. Nurses are required to be highly skilled in the forms of dialysis therapy as well as monitoring the patient's respiratory, cardiac, and hematologic systems. They must carefully monitor intake and output as well as any medications that the patient may be on while waiting for a potential kidney donor, which is the only cure for renal failure. Dialysis is not a cure and greatly affects the patient's quality of life, as many hours a week are spent making sure the toxins do not build up to too high a level. Infection can occur at the site where dialysis is performed, tubing can get detached and cause the patient to hemorrhage, or a clot can dislodge and cause death. Dialysis requires a team approach of nurses, social workers, primary care clinicians, nephrologists, and psychiatrists, who work together for the patient and their families. Mortality is higher for patients undergoing dialysis than for those receiving a kidney transplant. Survival rate on dialysis depends on the underlying disease process, and the overall 5-year survival rate is estimated to be about 36%.

Patients who have chronic or acute renal failure requiring dialysis are very sick patients.

> ## CLINICAL ALERT
>
> *Mortality rate for patients undergoing dialysis is high, and survival depends on the underlying disease process. The overall 5-year survival rate of patients undergoing dialysis is 36% and the most common cause of death is cardiac dysfunction. Without dialysis, these patients would die within days to weeks of kidney failure. Nurses provide emotional support to those undergoing dialysis understanding the chance of death without transplantation, and preparing patients and families.*

Renal Calculi

Calculi refer to stone formation within the urinary tract. Urinary crystals bind to form a nestlike structure, which grows to form a calculus (stone). Another term used for stone formation is lithiasis, and nephrolithiasis is stone formation in the kidney. Renal calculi can be asymptomatic or produce extremely painful colicky-type pain. The lifetime risk for men to develop a kidney stone is 20%, which is about 3 to 5 times greater than in women. Kidney stones are concentrated masses of crystallized substances such as calcium, oxalate, or uric acid that are excreted by the kidneys into the urine. The formation of calcium oxalate stone depends on the level of urinary supersaturation with calcium and oxalate. Approximately 70% of all diagnosed kidney stones consist of calcium oxalate crystals. More than half of all kidney stones are idiopathic; although urinary tract infection is a major predisposing factor, other factors include long-term use of antacids that contain calcium, hyperparathyroidism (cause of hypercalcemia), and high uric acid levels. Another type of kidney stone is the struvite stone, which typically form staghorn calculi in the renal pelvis and calyces and are large. These types of stones cause infections (e.g., Klebsiella, Proteus, and Pseudomonas), which leads to chronic kidney infections. Some diseases associated with nephrolithiasis are renal tube acidosis, gout, recurrent urinary tract infections, Crohn disease, prolonged immobilization, and laxative abuse. A family history of nephrolithiasis increases the risk for stone formation, which may suggest a hereditary metabolic disorder. A diet excessive in protein, oxalates, or calcium adds to the risk of developing kidney stones. The consumption of apple juice and grapefruit juice is associated with an increased risk, yet orange juice and lemon juice, which contain ample amount of citric acid, can help prevent kidney stones. Despite the fact that grapefruit juice contains citric acid, the reasons are unclear as to why it increases the risk of kidney stones. Pain is the hallmark of an acute episode, and when the stone moves to the ureters and trying to pass down toward the bladder, the pain is excruciating and begins in the costovertebral angle or flank. Nausea and vomiting may accompany the onset of the pain. There may be gross blood in the urine and sometimes clots. The pain may radiate from the flank to across the abdomen and into the labia in women and testicles in men. There may be urinary incontinence or dysuria, and the patient cannot feel comfortable because of the intense pain. The patient may also experience fever and chills with or without infection. Although renal calculi can be excruciatingly painful, they are not life-threatening.

Clinical Manifestations

Renal colic pain with acute onset, flank pain, microscopic or gross blood in the urine, nonspecific symptoms of nausea and vomiting, tachycardia, diaphoresis, low-grade fever with or without infection, frequent urination, and dysuria are commonly seen. In nonobstructing stones, in the renal calyces may be asymptomatic. There is tender renal angle or costovertebral tenderness.

Diagnostic Tests

Urinalysis for microscopic or gross blood; urine pH as normal is 5.9 and below 5.5 is suggestive of uric acid stones; midstream catch for microscopy and urine and sensitivity; Blood for urea, creatinine, electrolytes, calcium and urate, CT scan of abdomen and pelvis; x-ray of kidney, ureters, and bladder (KUB); and IVP confirm diagnosis.

Treatment

Treatment is aimed at pain relief, intravenous (IV) therapy, and antibiotics if necessary. Seventy-five percent of patients treated conservatively pass the stone therapy and antibiotics if necessary. Encourage frequent hydration. Stones should be sent to pathology to determine their composition, which would reveal what dietary changes if any are needed to prevent further stone formation. If a stone does not pass on its own, a procedure is aimed at breaking up the stone to small particles so that they will pass easily. This procedure is called lithotripsy, which uses extracorporeal shock-waves or laser to break up the stone, and for this the patient requires anesthesia. If the patient is septic or there is renal obstruction, there may be endoscopic placement of a retrograde stent and placement of a nephrostomy tube. Surgical intervention may be necessary if the stone persists with the other treatments.

Nursing Implications and Complications

Nurses must explain to the patient that vigorous fluid therapy keeping urine dilute will decrease further stone formation; depending on the type of stone, the patient must be educated on diet low in oxalate if stones are found to be oxylate, and also to avoid apple juice and grapefruit juice; if stones are calcium or other composition an underlying cause should be explored, such as a parathyroid problem; calcium stones are often treated with thiazides, which decrease urinary calcium excretion and has been found effective in preventing recurring stones; treat infections that occur with struvite calculi. Prepare the patient for any procedure such as lithotripsy or for a stent if stone is too large to be passed (stone less than 0.5 cm wide may pass spontaneously); assess patients for blockage of stone and possible urinary problems; manage the patient's severe pain and provide as much comfort as possible; strain all urine and give strains to patients who are at home (to know the composition of the stone for determining the medical management); and monitor pH of urine. Nurses in the hospital should ambulate patients frequently, and patients who are seen in offices should be instructed to ambulate often as immobility leads to stone formation.

CLINICAL ALERT

A kidney stone may block the flow of urine and cause urinary obstruction, which can lead to pyelonephritis. Nurses must assess urinary flow and if impaired they may necessitate immediate treatment for stone removal. Intractable pain can also occur and must be treated in a hospital setting.

Urinary Tract Infection

Urinary tract infections occur in both women and men although it is more common in women. It is the most common of all bacterial infection in women as the anatomy of women with the rectum in proximity to the urethra lends itself to ascending infections. Bacteria from the rectum or colonization in the vagina can ascend through the urethra into the bladder, causing a bladder infection or may ascend to the kidneys and cause pyelonephritis. A woman has a relatively short urethra, and sexual intercourse and use of condoms or spermicides can lead to infection. 30% of those with sustained bladder infections result in infection in the kidney. The most common are symptomatic bacteremia in the form of cystitis and pyelonephritis which produces fever, flank pain, and systemic symptoms. Some women do not adequately empty their bladders and the urine can back up causing infection. This is called vesicoureteral reflux, which can occur in patients with a long history of UTI's, and if it occurs during pregnancy there is an increased rate of fetal complications. The most common organisms that cause UTI's are *Escherichia coli, Trichomonas, Candida albicans, Chlamydia,* and *Enterobacteriaceae* in postmenopausal women.

Urinary tract infections in young men are rare but increase with age, and at age 65 UTI's are equal to that of women. If it occurs in young men it is usually as a result of bladder catheterization or surgery. As men age, the prostate gland enlarges, which leads to bladder outflow obstruction and residual urine builds up and pathogenic organisms grow. Men can also develop prostatitis, which is inflammation of the prostate gland due to infection and can be very painful. Despite the prevalence of these organisms, most men remain asymptomatic and are at a low risk of serious complications. If signs of failure to thrive or a worsening mental status is observed a gram-negative organism from a urinary tract infection can be life-threatening. Catheters and urinary or fecal incontinence are factors that can result in UTI's. Some men get UTI's as a result of having intercourse with a colonized partner. The organisms that infect men are *E. coli,* Proteus, Pseudomonas, Enterococcus, and coagulase-negative staphylococci.

Clinical Manifestations

UTI's cause the following symptoms: urinary frequency, urgency, hesitancy, dysuria, blood in the urine, and lower abdominal pain or feeling of pressure. If infection reaches the kidney then pyelonephritis occurs, causing flank pain (demonstrated by costovertebral angle tenderness [CVA]) during palpation, fever, and sometimes nausea and vomiting. The symptoms can be severe enough as to cause the person to go immediately to their healthcare provider's office or the emergency department to obtain relief.

Diagnostic Tests

Urine dipstick is performed to determine the presence of blood, white cells, nitrates, or protein; a culture and sensitivity is sent out to determine the organism responsible for the infection, so the patient is treated with the appropriate antimicrobial medication; ultrasonography may be ordered to evaluate for stones and view the kidneys; cystoscopy (viewing inside of the bladder); BUN, and creatinine test to evaluate renal function; urodynamic studies, which will determine adequate urinary flow and determine if residual urine is a problem; and IVP.

Treatment

Treatment is aimed at treating the responsible organism. Medications such as nitrofurantoin (Macrobid) treat many causes of urinary tract infections. The most common organism responsible for a large number of infections is *E. coli*. Some other antimicrobials used to treat UTIs are trimethoprim–sulfamethoxazole (Bactrim), broad-spectrum fluoroquinolone antibiotic (Cipro), and first-generation cephalosporin antibiotic (Keflex). Some women who suffer from frequent UTIs can be prescribed low-dose nitrofurantoin (Macrodantin) to take after intercourse.

Nursing Interventions and Complications

Nurses observe the signs and symptoms of UTIs and treat with the appropriate antibiotics based on the urine culture and sensitivity. Frequent urination acts as an antiseptic and prevents UTI, so nurses should educate patients on adequate hydration and frequent urination and spending time to empty the bladder completely. They also instruct the female patients to make sure with each urination or bowel movement they wipe from front to back. Once a woman has one urinary tract infection, she is very susceptible to getting more, so hygiene is enforced. Nurses also instruct women to urinate after sexual intercourse. Encourage hydration and drinking lots of water and drinking cranberry juice. When patients are hospitalized and require catheters, meticulous sterility must be maintained, and frequent hand washing is most important as well as cleaning incontinence patients to avoid infection. The complications are death in compromised patients in the hospital who develop a urinary infection.

CLINICAL ALERT

The complications are death in compromised patients in the hospital who develop a urinary infection. Persistent bacteria presence can result in septicemia in the very ill. Patients who require long-term indwelling urinary catheters are at the greatest risk. Nurses must maintain sterility in inserting Foley catheters and maintain excellent hygiene.

Interstitial Cystitis

Interstitial cystitis (IC) is a chronic syndrome of the lower urinary tract characterized by severe irritation when voiding and pelvic pain although the urine is sterile and cytologic tests are negative. Although the number of people suffering with IC is relatively low, it is felt that women suffering with urethral syndrome, urgency-frequency syndrome, recurrent infection, and chronic pelvic pain are misdiagnosed and may be having undiagnosed IC. Men with chronic nonbacterial prostatitis or pain may also have IC. Further, IC is associated with complex symptoms of urinary frequency with small voids, dysuria, nocturia, urinary urgency, suprapubic/pelvic/perineal pain, and dyspareunia (painful intercourse). The syndrome is characterized by periods of exacerbations and remissions, and symptoms become worse with stress. The premenstrual phase of a woman's cycle; after sexual intercourse; and after ingestion of acidic, alcoholic, spicy, caffeinated, and carbonated products are also associated with IC. Some associated conditions of patients with IC are irritable bowel syndrome, allergies, fibromyalgia, migraines, endometriosis, and vaginal pain disorders. Both males and females suffer with IC, but it mostly involves women with a mean age of 40.

Cystoscopy is really the only way to view the inside of the bladder and often nonspecific inflammation is found, but if petechial hemorrhages are distributed throughout the bladder and the bladder has a small capacity, then IC is diagnosed. Often, IC is diagnosed on the basis of the symptoms experienced with negative urine findings.

Clinical Manifestations

Pain increases as the bladder fills and there is some relief after urination; urgency; frequency; nocturia (awakening at night to urinate, sometimes several times); suprapubic discomfort; pelvic/perineal/anterior vaginal wall pain; symptoms are chronic although some periods are worse and there are some remissions; symptoms are unrelieved by antibiotics; and there is negative urine culture and cytologic test results.

Diagnostic Tests

Urinalysis, urine culture and sensitivity, cytology, urodynamic testing (to assess bladder sensation and to exclude detrusor muscle instability (muscle of urinary bladder that if unstable can cause urinary incontinence), vaginal and cervical cultures, potassium sensitivity test (if pain or urgency occurs, the test is positive and strongly correlates with IC), and cystoscopy (viewing inside the bladder) are utilized for diagnosis.

Treatment

The current treatment of IC is pentosan polysulfate sodium (Elmiron) three times a day, which reduces the bladder pain and discomfort of IC. Other treatment can be the use of nonsteroidal antiinflammatory drugs (NSAIDs), and Tums to buffer acidic urine. Occasionally, transcutaneous electrical nerve stimulation (TENS) is used based on the gate theory of pain in which an overstimulation of the nervous system modifies the perception of pain. Other drugs such as amitriptyline 10–75 mg daily or some of the calcium channel blockers, such as nifedipine, are used. Surgical intervention may be used to stretch the capacity of the bladder and as a last resort and may require a total cystectomy (removal of bladder) with urinary diversion.

Nursing Implications and Complications

Nursing care should be aimed at supporting these patients with a chronic disorder and to provide counseling, as stress and anxiety can increase symptoms, teach the patient to avoid liquids or food that may exacerbate the symptoms, as many patients are not aware of a dietary correlation (e.g., caffeine, chocolate, citrus fruits, tomatoes, carbonated drinks, spicy or acid foods). Explain that compliance with medication will help with symptoms, and the use of NSAIDs may provide more comfort. In very severe cases in which no relief is achieved, surgery may be required to destroy the nerves of the bladder or remove most of the diseased bladder and replace with healthy bowel, but those who require this drastic measure are only 1%–2% of those patients with IC.

CLINICAL ALERT

This is not a life-threatening disorder but may greatly affect one's quality of life. If surgery is required for unrelenting symptoms, the nurse provides pre and post care as well as continued emotional support as the surgery may require removal of the bladder and alteration of the urination process (such as suprapubically).

Glomerulonephritis

Acute glomerulonephritis most commonly presents after infection of the skin, pharynx, and certain strains of group A (B hemolytic) streptococcus, but other causes can be systemic lupus erythematosus, vascular injury (hypertension), diabetes, and disseminated intravascular coagulation. Because of the infection, there is an antigen-antibody reaction leading to the formation of an insoluble immune complex that becomes trapped in the glomeruli (part of kidney responsible for filtration). Many glomeruli become blocked by this inflammatory reaction, and those glomeruli that are blocked become excessively permeable, which then allows both protein and red blood cells to leak into the urine but with retention of metabolic wastes, sodium, and water. Glomerulonephritis in severe cases can lead to partial or complete renal shutdown. The acute inflammation of the glomeruli usually subsides in about 2 weeks and in most cases the kidneys return to normal functioning within the next few weeks or months. Sometimes, however, if many glomeruli are destroyed beyond repair, a small number of patients may progress to chronic glomerulonephritis, which results in chronic renal failure. Glomerulonephritis is three times more common in males. Complaints initially are shortness of breath, headache, weakness, anorexia, and flank pain. Proteinuria, hematuria, and azotemia (increased nitrogenous waste) is also present. Patients become edematous (face and lower extremities) and develop hypertension.

Acute glomerulonephritis may follow an acute illness, but most persons who develop chronic glomerulonephritis have no history of infection, which suggests that this form of the disease may result from an immunologic mechanism. The course of the chronic disease is extremely variable, where some patients feel well while others progress to renal failure, resulting in end-stage renal disease.

Clinical Manifestations

Edema (facial, orbital, lower extremities), hypertension, shortness of breath, generalized malaise, flank pain, smoky or coffee-colored urine, decreased urination, and nausea are some of the signs.

Diagnostic Tests

Urinalysis with attention to sediment, electrolytes, BUN, creatinine, CBC, anti-streptolysin O titer (aids in the diagnosis of conditions with streptoccocal infections), 24-hour urine collection for protein and creatinine, serum protein levels (decreased in glomerulonephritis), serum calcium (decreased), sedimentation rate (inflammatory and necrotic processes that cause alteration in proteins, causing aggregation of heavier RBCs that fall to the bottom), KUB, renal sonogram, and renal biopsy will confirm the diagnosis.

Treatment

Treatment is aimed at symptoms, such as diuretic for salt retention and edema; if hyperkalemia, treat with Kayexalate; oxygen for pulmonary edema; and if infection is present, treat with antibiotics. Corticosteroids may also be used to decrease antibody synthesis and decrease inflammation, and vasodilators are used for elevated blood pressure. Dialysis possibly may be needed.

Nursing Interventions and Complications

Excessive fluid volume due to edema and sodium retention causes the nurse to monitor input and output and restrict dietary sodium, weigh patient daily, and assess for any signs and symptoms of fluid overload. There is a risk for infection as the patient has a decreased immune response, and so the nurse must monitor vital signs and temperature often and get cultures when any infection is suspected. The patient may not have an understanding of glomerulonephritis and the nurse educates him on the disease and any tests that are being done. The nurse should monitor lab work and report any abnormality or change in finding. The patient may have anxiety or difficulty coping with the diagnosis, and the nurse should support the patient if on bedrest and encourage verbalization and when blood pressure, edema, and sedimentation rate are reduced, the patient should be ambulated. The nurse should monitor any medications ordered and administer to patient and explain to the patient the purpose of the medications. Discharge instruction should include how frequently the patient should see their health care provider because the nurse knows recovery of acute glomerulonephritis can take up to 2 years. Educate all patients on prevention, including getting prompt treatment with antibiotics for any streptococcus-related illness or any acute illness.

CLINICAL ALERT

Complications can result depending on the amount of glomeruli damaged. In chronic glomerulonephritis, progression of renal deterioration may be slow or rapid, which can result in complete renal failure requiring dialysis and require kidney transplant if the patient is a candidate for a transplant. Nurses assess all the symptoms of patients with glomerulonephritis, especially urinary function, respiratory status, fluid balance, nutrition, skin care of edematous tissue, and prevention of infections.

Renal Failure

Chronic renal failure results from an irreversible loss of large numbers of functioning nephrons (the functioning unit of the kidney, and there are approximately 1 million nephrons in each kidney). Chronic renal failure can result from glomerular, vascular, or tubular disease. Congenital anomalies (e.g., polycystic kidney disease), infection, and obstructive disease of the urinary system can all lead to renal insufficiency. A characteristic of most forms of chronic renal failure is that there is progressive deterioration of kidney function long after the initial insult is present. Chronic renal failure results in disturbances in electrolyte and fluid balance, elimination of metabolic wastes and toxins, erythropoietin production and blood pressure control. The severity of the progression of chronic renal failure depends on the number of nephrons damaged, as healthy nephrons can compensate for the destroyed ones by enlarging, which increases their clearance capacity, but eventually they become sclerotic and cease to function as well. The kidneys in chronic renal failure can function until approximately 70% of nephrons are destroyed. When this occurs, the patient needs dialysis or a transplanted kidney to survive. Chronic kidney disease disproportionately affects African Americans compared to other ethnic groups.

Acute renal failure is a common clinical syndrome and is defined as an abrupt decline of renal function. There is a decline in the GFR and the kidneys lose their ability to excrete toxic metabolic wastes. The BUN and creatinine rises and the patient can go from normal uremic functioning to uremia in a week. Most forms of acute renal failure are reversible if correct diagnosis is made. A decline in renal perfusion caused by a myocardial infarction, hypotension, sepsis, shock, peritonitis, and extracellular volume depletion can cause acute renal failure. Hospitalized patients, who are taking nephrotoxic medications, have had surgery: liver or heart failure, disseminated intravascular coagulation (DIC), hemorrhage, burns, trauma, or hypovolemic shock may result in acute renal failure.

In the healthy individual, potassium is exchanged in the nephrons for either sodium or hydrogen ion and therefore can conserve potassium, but when the nephrons are not functioning there is no way to remove the potassium and hyperkalemia develops. High levels develop that are not compatible with cardiac functioning. The loss of sodium leads to hyponatremia, and when the hydrogen ion is excreted acidosis develops. Because the metabolic wastes cannot be excreted, BUN and creatinine rise, neurologic symptoms such as confusion, convulsions, and coma develop. If conservative measures such as diuretics, low-protein diet, and electrolyte management do not work, then dialysis is required.

Both chronic and acute renal failures pose serious alterations in the physiologic functioning of the patient who may require dialysis and the only alternative is a renal transplant.

Clinical Manifestations

Anorexia, weakness, fatigue, pruritus, nausea, shortness of breath (fluid overload), edema, hypertension, drowsiness, lethargy, and uremia (buildup of nitrogenous wastes), oliguria, and cardiac problems due to hyperkalemia are generally observed.

Diagnostic Tests

BUN and creatinine levels, potassium level, electrocardiogram (to determine cardiac changes with hypokalemia), sodium level, arterial blood gases, urinalysis, CBC (anemia due to loss of erythropoietin), renal sonogram, and Doppler flow study (to rule out renal artery stenosis/thrombosis) are performed to ensure correct diagnosis.

Treatment

Treatment depends on the underlying cause. If the cause is hypovolemia, the treatment is with hypotonic IV solutions such as 0.45% saline. If the cause of the renal failure is nephrotoxic drugs, treat with agents that increase renal blood flow such as mannitol or loop diuretics. When medications fail to treat the renal failure, dialysis is required. Dietary management is most important and must include collaboration among nurses, dieticians, and physicians.

Nursing Management and Complications

Deficient/excess fluid should be monitored for edema and weigh patient each day. In case of imbalanced nutrition, decrease protein in diet but increase carbohydrates and fats. Safety is important as the patient may be confused; therefore, reorient patient and assist out of bed. Assess for signs of bleeding and prevent infection; monitor lab values. Ineffective coping and deficient knowledge are diagnoses that require the nurse to address supportive emotional care and explain all that is happening to the patient and any tests that are required. The complications of renal failure require lifelong dialysis, and in some cases death will occur if a renal transplantation is not an option.

CLINICAL ALERT

Kidney failure is one of the most significant causes of death and long-term disability as functioning kidneys are vital to maintain functions in the body that are needed to live. Nurses assess symptoms, lab values, and vital signs and if the patient is at the end stage the patient and family are included in the plan for the patient. Emotional care is given at the end of life.

CASE STUDY

Mary Q. is a 42-year-old woman who has been relatively healthy most of her life, with few complaints other than the occasional muscle soreness due to working out every day. Over the last several months, she has had pelvic pain and a feeling of pressure that is somewhat relieved by urination. She has had several episodes of urinary tract infection in the past, but she says "this is different," and the symptoms she is experiencing are becoming chronic. She sees her internist, and a urine culture and sensitivity as well as a urine for cytology are both negative. She is complaining that it is affecting her quality of life and is worried that the internist may think the discomfort is in her head. She has pain with intercourse and it is affecting her marriage. When asked about her diet, she likes spicy foods, diet soda, and coffee, but states she has always eaten and drank these items, and that she has recently enjoyed chocolate also. She denies any other problems when a review of systems is done by the internist. She is referred to a urologist, who does a urological workup and a cystoscopy.

QUESTIONS

1. What is this patient's most likely diagnosis?
2. What would the urologist use to decide on a diagnosis?
3. What is the nursing diagnosis and intervention that the nurse would initiate with this patient?
4. How would the nurse know that the patient was not experiencing another urinary tract infection?
5. What is the treatment that would help relieve symptoms for this patient?

Suggested Readings

Baker MJ, Longyhore DS. Dietary calcium, calcium supplements, and the risk of calcium oxalate kidney stones. *Am J Health Syst Pharm.* 2006;63(8):772-775.

Corall AH, Mulby AG. *Primary Care Medicine.* 4th ed. Philadelphia, PA: Lippincott Williams & Wilkins; 2000.

Doenges ME, Moorhouse MF, Murr AC. *Nursing Diagnosis Manual.* Philadelphia, PA: F.A. Davis; 2010.

Domino F. *The 5 Minute Clinical Consults 2011.* 19th ed. Philadelphia, PA: Wolters Kluwer/Lippincott Williams & Wilkins; 2010.

Goroll AH, Mulley AG. *Primary Care Medicine.* 4th ed. Philadelphia, PA: Lippincott Willaims & Wilkins; 2000.

Guyton AC, Hall JE. *Textbook of Medical Physiology.* 9th ed. Philadelphia, PA: W.B. Saunders; 1996.

Kelley WN. *Textbook of Internal Medicine.* 3rd ed. Philadelphia, PA: Lippincott-Raven; 1992.

McPhee SJ, Papadakis MA, Rabow MW. *2011 Current Medical Diagnosis & Treatment.* New York: McGraw-Hill; 2011.

Peters RM, Olsen KL. Kidney disease awareness among high-risk African Americans. *Am J Nurse Pract.* 2010;14(3):40-47.

Phipps WJ, Monhahan FD, Sands JK, Marek JF, Neighbors M. *Medical-Surgical Nursing Health and Illness Perspectives.* 7th ed. St. Louis, MO: Mosby; 2003.

Professional Guide to Signs and Symptoms. 5th ed. Philadelphia, PA: Lippincott Williams & Wilkins; 2009.

Star W, Lommel LL, Shannon MT. *Women's Primary Health Care Protocols for Practice.* 2nd ed. San Francisco, CA: UCSF Nursing Press; 2004.

Taber's Cyclopedic Medical Dictionary. Philadelphia, PA: F.A. Davis; 2009.

Wells KA. Nephrolithiasis with unusual initial symptoms. *J Manipulative Physiol Ther.* 2000;23(3):196-201.

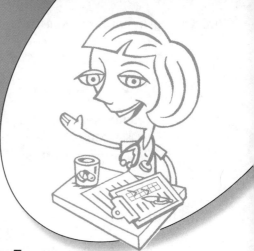

chapter 7

Musculoskeletal System

LEARNING OBJECTIVES

At the end of this chapter, the reader/student will be able to:

- Describe the pathophysiology of the bone diseases and bone degradation
- Compare the pathophysiology of osteomyelitis, osteoporosis, osteoarthritis, and rheumatoid arthritis
- Discuss and implement nursing measures in the management of musculoskeletal disorders

---

KEY WORDS

Osteomyelitis   Osteoarthritis
Osteoporosis   Rheumatoid Arthritis

Introduction

Bone disorders affect a great majority of patients. Of the diseases discussed here, many affect the older adult more than younger patients, with the exception of early-onset juvenile rheumatoid arthritis (not discussed here). Older adults often attribute bone pain, range-of-motion limitations, swelling, and other symptoms to the aging process. Because of these reasons, the nurse plays a significant role in patient education to include screening especially in the prevention of osteoporosis both in men and women. In addition, early assessments that include a physical assessment may elucidate range-of-motion abnormalities often attributed to old age. With the advent of awareness, especially in the field of rheumatoid arthritis and an aging population, prompt assessment is paramount.

Osteomyelitis

Osteomyelitis is an infection of the bone and its innermost structure: the marrow. Infections of the bone and marrow are classified as acute or chronic. Osteolytic infections occur when bone is exposed to granulomatous infections (tuberculosis) or when exposed to viral, fungal, or bacterial (pyogenic) infections.

Common bacterial bone infections involve *Staphylococcus aureus*, streptococci, *Escherichia coli*, gonococci, pneumococci, *Salmonella*, *Pseudomonas*, *Haemophilus influenzae*, and group B streptococci. Acute bone infections if not identified quickly can become chronic infections that are often difficult to treat, monitor, and manage.

Infectious agents reach the bone in various ways. There is hematogenous spread from systemic infections that spread via the bloodstream. Primary bone infections due to impairment of the bone structure and infections from surrounding organs/tissues also contribute to osteomyelitis. An open fracture or deep penetrating wound/trauma is an additional contributory factor. Gross inflammatory responses generate after exposure to infectious agents, causing polymorphonuclear leukocytes to aggregate. Because of the inflammatory response, local pressure on sensitive bone and surrounding tissues leads to edema formation. Pressure from edema potentiates ischemia and possible necrosis and bone death. And because of the tight structure, pus and bacteria can be pushed along the sensitive Volkmann canals, spreading infection.

In chronic osteomyelitis, constant inflammatory responses cause the development of granulomas tissue that eventually turns into scar tissue. Many times, this scar tissue sequestrates the infection. This is known as Brodie abscess. Additional overlay of bone continues to occur. Clinical manifestations such as chronic pain, edema, erythema, and warmth continue to perpetuate. Quality of life can be severely affected.

Clinical Manifestations

- Presence of constitutional symptoms: fever, chills, malaise, acutely ill
- Labs: erythrocyte sedimentation rate (ESR), white blood cell (WBC) elevation [leukocytes in particular]
- Pain (often refractory)
- Signs of the inflammatory response: edema, erythema, sensitivity, reduced range of motion of involved joint and surrounding areas
- Positive blood cultures (though not always positive)

Diagnostic Tests

Radiographic films may not always demonstrate an active infection and, oftentimes, changes to the joint may not be present until 10–14 days after infection sets in. At this point, extensive bone/joint destruction might have already occurred.

Magnetic resonance imaging demonstrates intraosseous and extraosseous changes before they are seen on radiographic films. At times, bone biopsy and/or wound cultures will be necessary.

Treatment

Treatment for osteomyelitis is long-term. Empiric use of antibiotics is required and in some cases, if the osteomyelitis is occurring along the spine, spinal decompression may be necessary.

Antibiotic use is dependent on the pathogen causing the infection. At the very least, patients will be on a 2-week course of intravenous antibiotics followed by a 4- to 8-week course of oral antibiotics. For refractory infections, insertion of a peripheral inserted central catheter (PICC) line for longer-term antibiotics will be required. The PICC lines are inserted before the patient leaves the hospital and can be inserted by specialty-trained registered nurses or physicians. Chronic infections require about 8–10 weeks of therapy. Common antibiotics include piperacillin-tazobactam, ampicillin- sulbactam, or ticarcillin-clavulanate. If the patient is allergic to penicillin, clindamycin or metronidazole is used.

Nursing Interventions and Complications

Nursing interventions should concern managing, monitoring therapeutic modalities ordered for the patient. In addition, the nurse should provide support and protect the bone from further injury. It is important that the nurse encourage that the patient verbalize what he or she feels as the condition is painful, limiting in terms of function, and that treatments are long-lasting. The patient should also be encouraged to be as independent as possible.

To protect the integrity of the infection, nurses should use aseptic technique when changing dressings. Hand washing prior to dressing changes is necessary. Wounds should be irrigated well and appropriately. Because healing also occurs from the inside out, nurses should encourage patients to eat a nutritious diet rich in protein for wound synthesis. Vitamin C should be supplemented. Management and vigilance of pain is the primary concern for nurses. Further, because acute osteomyelitis often converts to chronic disease, new-onset pain, or pain that is refractory to treatment, should be promptly reported.

Patients should be repositioned often especially if there are strictures such as a cast. Skin integrity must be maintained and protected to prevent secondary infections as well as further skin breakdown. If the patient is going for other diagnostic procedures, it is the responsibility of the nurse to fully explain the tests and procedures in order to help reduce anxiety.

CLINICAL ALERT

Persistent pain or pain that is refractory to medication should be promptly reported. Pain not only alters the integrity of the healing process but it is also a hallmark that secondary infections may occur. Changes in the patient's vital signs and prompt wound assessments with timely reporting of changes wards off further infection spread.

Osteoporosis

As the patient ages, significant changes to bone parenchyma occur. The degeneration of bone cause significant bone abnormalities and bone/joint-related pain. Osteopenia, which is the term used to define the beginnings of bone changes, often heralds bone discomfort and limitations in movement.

According to the World Health Organization, bone mass density that is 1–2.5 standard deviations below the normal values are considered to indicate low bone mass (osteopenia) (www.who.int/chp/topics/Osteoporosis.pdf). Osteoporosis occurs when bone densities are more than 2.5 standard deviations less than the normal values.

Osteoporosis can be classified into three broad categories: type I, postmenopausal; type II, senile; and type III, secondary. Type III can occur at any age, types I and II begin to appear at or around ages 50–70 years, with senile or type II being more pronounced among the very old and fragile patient. Type I is commonly seen in the postmenopausal female and is primarily due to the reduction of the bone protector: estrogen. Because bone generation is a complex process of reabsorption and bone genesis, estrogen, though poorly understood, interferes with the bone genesis cycle. Type II osteoporosis is found among both genders. Affecting men and women aged >70 years, bone loss and mineral wasting potential weaken bone matrix. A slow decline is common after age 40 years. If the patient has contributory risk factors, bone loss is more pronounced. Bone loss for both genders is approximately 3% per decade of life. Type III is risk factor–based. Diseases, genetics, medications, and lifestyle are important secondary factors to type III osteoporosis. Therefore, assessing the patient for additional factors must be considered. These factors include important risk factors: advancing age, genetics, lifestyle (smoking, alcohol use), nutritional factors, small frame, being female, disease process (diabetes, rheumatoid arthritis), anemia, Cushing syndrome, malabsorption syndromes (calcium deficiency, vitamin D deficiency, diets high in protein), and psycho-neuroendocrinology disorders such as bulimia or anorexia nervosa. Medication usage also may contribute to bone degeneration: thyroid hormone replacements, steroids, chemotherapy, diuretics, long-term lithium therapy, heparin, and seizure medications.

In all three types of osteoporosis, there is progressive lifelong bone matrix destruction as well as an increased risk for fractures of the spine, hip, pelvis, and humerus.

Clinical Manifestations

- A skeletal fracture: common sites—hip, pelvis, and humerus
- Sudden fractures or pathologic fractures
- Falls
- Weakness
- Anorexia
- Changes in gait/balance
- Pain

Diagnostic Tests

The gold standard is the bone density test. Known as the dual-energy x-ray absorptiometry (DEXA) scan, an analysis is made of the hip and spine. The DEXA scan measures bone mass density (BMD). Serial height measurements can also be part of the diagnostic process. Serum levels of calcium, albumin, electrolytes, complete blood count, and thyroid levels are also important for diagnostic purposes.

Treatment

In osteopenic bones, oral calcium and vitamin D supplementation should commence as soon as the bone mass density indicates. For osteoporosis, bisphosphonates are common medications. They include alendronate, risedronate, and ibandronate. Raloxifene is an excellent hormonal replacement modulator for osteoporosis. Inhaled calcitonin is another choice and it has demonstrated a reduction in fractures among postmenopausal females.

Nursing Interventions and Complications

The nurse's focus on the care of the patient with osteoporosis should center on fracture prevention, safety, monitoring for therapeutic and adverse effects of medications, and screening, monitoring, and patient education.

In addition, pain management is important especially in the presence of a fracture. Physical therapy and/or occupational therapy referrals are important in order to prevent muscle atrophy, excessive pain, and to improve overall strength. Nurses should encourage their patients to be as independent as possible and be active in mild to moderate weight-bearing exercises as tolerated. Patient education should include diagnostic testing after age 50 years. According to the U.S. Preventive Services Task force (USPSTF), a DEXA scan is recommended after age 65 for women and age 70 for men.

Medication education is also paramount, as some of the medications require injections and oral administration. Some medications instruct patients that they cannot lay down for approximately ½ to 1 hour postadministration.

CLINICAL ALERT

Fracture prevention is a priority among osteoporotic patients. Considering the associated iatrogenic consequence of weak bones, which includes falls, the nurse plays an instrumental role in its prevention. Screening patients with known risk factors is an integral function of the registered nurse as is patient education.

Osteoarthritis

Arthritis is the degeneration of joints. It is a noninflammatory disease that affects both genders equally. The aging adult attributes aches and pains to the aging process, but in many cases, the pain is linked to joint degradation. There are two broad classifications of osteoarthritis: primary, where the cause in unknown, and secondary, when there is a known contributory factor to joint destruction.

In osteoarthritis, cartilage and subchondral bone are lost. Excessive osteophytes are formed and concentrated around the disturbed joint. Surrounding aspects of the joints are also affected by osteoarthritis. Ligaments, muscles, and tendons as well as the cushioning function of the synovial fluid are disturbed. Osteoarthritis is a classic example of joint wear and tear. And unlike its cousin, rheumatoid arthritis, joint destruction is limited to the joints and it does not have the component of additional systemic manifestations.

Osteoarthritis can be compared to the peeling of a banana peel. When the outermost layer, the articular cartilage, is removed, the meat of the bone (collagen structure) is exposed. When exposed, the collagen peels, fractures, frays, fissures, or erodes. Under wear and tear, cracks develop, synovial fluid leaks, and bone-to-bone surfaces interface. As true with any form of body destruction, inflammatory responses automatically occur. In osteoarthritis, the inflammatory response causes the development of subchondral cysts. These cysts limit movement, produce pain, and decrease joint size (Figure 7–1).

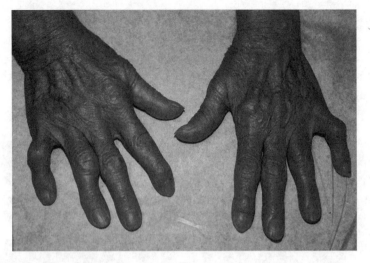

FIGURE 7–1 • Bony enlargement of most distal interphalangeal (DIP) and proximal interphalangeal (PIP) joints consistent with Heberden and Bouchard nodes. (Reproduced with permission from Usatine RP, et al. *The Color Atlas of Family Medicine*. New York: McGraw-Hill; 2009, figure 91-1. Courtesy of Richard P. Usatine, MD.)

Clinical Manifestations

- Pain, dull in nature or may be sharp, limited to the affected joint and immediate surrounding areas. Pain is usually on a unilateral side, and commonly affected joints include the hands, wrists, foot, hips, knees, and spine (cervical and/or lumbar)
- Range-of-motion pain limitation
- Stiffness
- Joint instability: falls, gait disturbance, and balance problems
- Crepitus
- Joint effusions
- Muscle wasting/atrophy
- Development of Heberden nodes (found on the proximal interphalangeal joints) and Bouchard nodes (found on the fingers)

Diagnostic Tests

There are no specific tests to determine joint damage. However, radiographic pictures can demonstrate joint damage that has occurred. On x-ray, joint narrowing may be seen. Laboratory assessments include ESR, complete blood counts with differentials, and electrolytes.

Treatment

Treatments are geared at symptom management. Analgesics taken orally often include nonsteroidal anti-inflammatory drugs (NSAIDs). Medications such as Advil, ibuprofen, and naproxen control the inflammatory aspect of osteoarthritis and are also good agents for pain management. Topical agents can be applied directly to the affected joint and are useful in that there is a significant decrease in the incidence of systemic absorption, a good choice for an elderly person.

Nurses are instrumental at considering physical therapy consults for patients who require assistance in gait, balance, and overall strengthening for fall prevention, keeping in mind that stronger bones can significantly reduce the incidence of falls.

Injections directly into the joint structure also provide pain relief, often for long periods of time. Administration of injections can also assist with pain relief that allows for physical therapy, which in turns strengths the structure. Types of injections include steroids (aimed at reducing inflammation) or injections of hyaluronic acid which helps lubricate the joint, reducing the caustic joint surface contact.

If symptom management is unattainable, surgery is considered. Surgery involves joint replacement (arthroplasty), osteotomy, or arthroscopic surgery of the knee joint. As with any surgery, special consideration must be given to the patient with advancing age, comorbidities, functional stressors, medication use, and cardiopulmonary status.

Nursing Interventions and Complications

Focus on pain management is paramount. Promptly assessing, evaluating, and administration of pain medication is the nurse's priority. Pain assessment helps not only reduce pain but also assess if pain medications are achieving the desired therapeutic effect. The patient will have an overall sense of well-being and of being in control of a destructive disease process. Therefore, encouraging the verbalization of feelings is critical. Encourage the use of assistive devices such as canes, crutches, braces, or a walker. If the patient is wearing an assistive device that may cause skin irritation, watch for skin irritations.

CLINICAL ALERT

As with all bone diseases, limitations in movement place the patient at risk for falls. With the osteoarthritic patient, encouragement of the use of assistive devices decreases the fall risk tremendously.

Rheumatoid Arthritis

As with osteoarthritis, rheumatoid arthritis is a joint degradation disease. Unlike osteoarthritis, joint degradation is symmetrical. There is also a strong degree of associated systemic manifestations not seen in osteoarthritis.

Rheumatoid arthritis is an autoimmune destructive disease in that the body auto-destructs itself, targeting joints and their surrounding supports.

An infectious process starts off the cascade. Synovial fluid lymphocytes herald the initiation of immunoglobulin G (IgG), which are foreign in nature. IgG and IgM anti-immunoglobulins result. These factors dictate the rheumatoid factor (RF) and it is identified in serum. A complex cascade ensues that leads to joint destruction.

Joint destruction is persistent and systemic. Joint effusions are prevalent. The formation of fibrin clots and newly formed granulation tissue take up the joint space, eventually eroding the remaining joint/bone. Pannus develops (a thickened synovial joint fluid). Pannus potentiates the development of ankylosis (joint fusion). Basic criteria for rheumatoid arthritis are stiffness, more pronounced in the morning (longer than 1 hour); three or more affected joints; arthritis in the hands; symmetrical joint involvement; the presence of nodules, a positive RF; and changes to joints on x-ray.

As it is a systemic disease, general constitutional systems are also present (Figures 7–2 and 7–3).

Clinical Manifestations

- Progressive symmetrical joint pain: at rest and at night
- Depression
- Fever, often low-grade
- Erythema, stiffness, and warmth of the involved joints
- Presence of rheumatoid arthritis nodules
- Fixed flexion of the smaller hand joints: swan neck and boutonniere
- Decreased or limited range of motion
- Hand muscle atrophy
- Other organ involvement: pleural effusions, pericarditis, nephropathy, eye/vision changes, vasculitis, lymphadenopathy, and splenomegaly

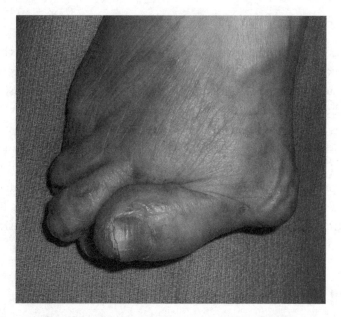

FIGURE 7–2 • Deviation at the metatarsalphalangeal joints from bony destruction in advanced rheumatoid arthritis. (Reproduced with permission from Usatine RP, et al. *The Color Atlas of Family Medicine*. New York: McGraw-Hill; 2009, figure 92-3. Courtesy of Richard P. Usatine, MD.)

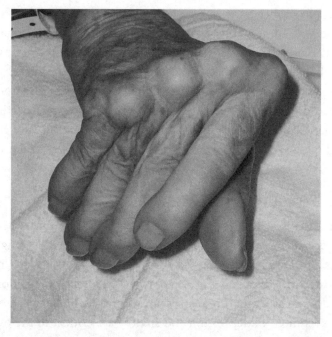

FIGURE 7–3 • Ulnar deviation at metacarpophalangeal joints seen in a 79-year-old woman with advanced rheumatoid arthritis. (Reproduced with permission from Usatine RP, et al. *The Color Atlas of Family Medicine*. New York: McGraw-Hill; 2009, figure 92-4. Courtesy of Kelly Foster, MD.)

Diagnostic Tests

Patient assessment utilizing the latest criteria for classification of rheumatoid arthritis according to the 2010 Rheumatoid Arthritis Classification Criteria, An American College of Rheumatology/European League Against Rheumatism: Collaborative Initiative.

Diagnosis is difficult because joint destruction and its associated changes are often not visible until late disease. Laboratory workup should include rheumatoid factor (RF), anti-cyclic citrullinated peptide (anti-CCP) antibodies, and C-reactive protein (CRP). Synovial fluid aspiration may be indicated but it is not the sole indicator for rheumatoid arthritis. Radiologic findings in late disease, as with osteoarthritis, will demonstrate joint destruction, effusion, and/or pannus formation.

Treatment

Goals of treatment are focused on pain reduction, limiting the effects the disease has on mobility, preventing falls/fractures, and educating the patient.

The nurse plays an important role because the patient must be educated on disease etiology and progression as well as treatments that are centered on medications, physical therapy, and rest.

The nurse will administer NSAIDs that include cyclo-oxygenase (COX) inhibitors keeping in mind, as with osteoarthritis, gastrointestinal (GI) disturbances and bleeding/ulcer risks. The nurse may also administer a selective group of medications known as DMARDS. DMARDS are disease-modifying antirheumatic drugs and the drug of choice is methotrexate. Additional medications are corticoid steroids that assist with inflammation, and biologic response-modifying agents such as etanercept, infliximab, and adalimumab.

Nursing Interventions and Complications

Patient education is central as this is a destructive autoimmune-mediated disease. Patients need to understand that they did not do anything wrong to develop this autoimmune disorder, so verbalization of feelings are important.

As with osteoarthritis, concepts of mobilization, safety, medications, and use of assistive devices are signature instructions from the nurse.

Prompt assessment of depression and anxiety are critical to the overall well-being of the patient.

CLINICAL ALERT

Prevention of further joint destruction is key. Because rheumatoid arthritis may not be known until progressive joint damage has occurred, focusing on coping mechanisms and fall prevention due to weak joints are necessary. Body image disturbance should be addressed by the nurse as well.

CASE STUDY: RHEUMATOID ARTHRITIS

A 36-year-old female Caucasian patient presents with a 1-year history of symmetrical arthritic pain in both joints of the hands. On assessment, it is noted that the hands are distorted in shape (swan shaped, ulnar deviation), are warm to touch, and edematous. The patient states that on awakening, the joints are very stiff and painful but that the stiffness and pain lessen as the day wears on. Also noted are nodes (Heberden nodes) on the distal metacarpal joints. All laboratory results are within normal ranges as are her urinalysis, liver function, and renal tests.

QUESTIONS

1. Following the guidelines for the diagnosis of rheumatoid arthritis, what would be the expected additional workup for this patient?
2. Should the patient be referred to a specialist and, if yes, to whom?
3. Should the primary care provider commence any noninflammatory medications at this point?
4. What other medications would the patient be started on?
5. What side effects, adverse effects, and therapeutic effects should the nurse monitor?
6. Are there any extraarticular symptoms that the nurse should assess and monitor? And if yes, what would they be?

REVIEW QUESTIONS

1. **The nurse is providing patient teaching. The patient asks the nurse what is the difference between osteoarthritis and rheumatoid arthritis. Choose the best response by the nurse.**

   A. Both diseases involve bilateral joint swelling

   B. One has a local presentation, the other a systemic presentation

   C. Both are caused because of an autoimmune response

   D. One has erythemic painful joints, the other has cyanotic painful joints

2. **The patient has been newly diagnosed with osteomyelitis. After a course of IV antibiotics in an inpatient setting, the patient will be discharged to home on continued IV antibiotics for three months via a peripherally inserted central catheter (PICC) line. In order of priority, what is the first patient teaching focus of the nurse?**

   A. Administer your antibiotics on time everyday

   B. Call the visiting nurse if the PICC line is tender

   C. Follow-up with your provider in 2 weeks as instructed

   D. Wash your hands before administering your medications

3. **An elderly female patient asks why she has to go for a bone density test. She says she feels fine, walks every day, takes her calcium supplements, and there is no family history of osteoporosis in her family. Her past medical history is hypertension, hyperlipidemia, smoking 30 years × 1 ppd (pack per day) and obesity. What is the nurse's best response?**

   A. Screening is important for all postmenopausal patients

   B. Your BMI (body mass index) is >34

   C. Some of the medications may cause lethargy, so you might exercise as often

   D. There is a long history of nicotine exposure

Osteoarthritis vs. Rheumatoid Arthritis

Presentation	Osteoarthritis (OA)	Rheumatoid Arthritis (RA)
Systemic presentation	Not present	Dull pain, inflammation, frequent afternoon fatigue, ulner deviation, muscle atrophy, swelling of the knuckles, synovial thickness, depression
Duration/presentation of joint stiffness	Morning stiffness lasts <30 min, but stiffness returns later in the day worsening as the day progresses	Morning stiffness last longer >1 hour, worse in the AM
Effusions	Local inflammation/effusion sometimes	Common
Nodules	Herberden's & Bouchard's nodules	Same as OA, especially on extensor surfaces, swan neck deformity. Biopsy may be necessary to rule out gouty tophi
Associated symptoms	Bony enlargement, deformity, instability, restricted movement, joint locking, sleep disturbance, depression, bursitis, fibromyalgia, gout	Frequent feeling of "being sick inside," with fevers, weight loss, or involvement of other organ systems, carpal tunnel syndrome, extraarticular manifestations: nodules, vasculitis, pulmonary, cardiac, skin (vasculitis), Sjogen's syndrome, scleritis, Fetty syndrome
Severity	Less severe	More severe
Disease process	Normal wear and tear of joints	Chronic autoimmune
Treatment	NSAIDs	NSAIDs, DMARDs (methotrexate), anti-malarial (Plaquenil), eye drops
Gender	Common in both men and women. Before age 50: men > women, after age 50: women > men	Affects women more than men
Diagnosis	x-ray, pain assessment, pre-articular and articular source of pain, presence of deformity, evidence of muscle wasting, local inflammation, asymmetrical joints	Inflammatory markers: CRP & ESR Anemia (ferritin, TIBC, UIBC)
Pain with movement	Movement increases pain	Movement decreases pain

(continued)

Osteoarthritis vs. Rheumatoid Arthritis (*Continued*)

Presentation	Osteoarthritis (OA)	Rheumatoid Arthritis (RA)
Pattern of joints that are affected	Asymmetrical & may spread to the other side. Symptoms begin gradually and are often limited to one set of joints, usually the finger joints closest to the fingernails or the thumbs, large wearing joints	Symmetrical. Often affects small and large joints on both sides of the body such as both hands, both wrists or elbows or the balls of both feet
Age of onset	Most commonly occurs at >age 50	Usual age of onset 20–40 years of age
Speed of onset	Gradual, over many years	Rapid, within a year
Joint symptoms	Joints are painful but no swelling, affects joints symmetrically, and affects bigger joints such as hips and knees. Localized with variable, progressive course	Joints are painful, swollen, and stiff; affects joints symmetrically, affects smaller joints such as hands and ankles. Systemic with exacerbations and remissions
Clinical	One or several joints; enlarged, cool, and hard on palpation	Joints are swollen; red, warm, tender, and painful; several joints are involved
Radiologic findings	Loss of joint space and articular cartilage, routine wear and tear, osteophytes, sclerosis, cysts, loose bodies, alignment	Bony erosions, soft tissue swelling, angular deformities
Lab findings	Rheumatoid factor (RF) negative, transient elevation in ESR possible (due to synovitis)	RF positive, elevated ESR & CRP, presence of antinuclear antibody (ANA), arthrocentesis

Osteoarthritis vs Rheumatoid Arthritis.
Diffen LLC, 2013. Web. Thu Jul 18, 2013.
http://www.diffen.com/difference/Osteoarthritis_vs_Rheumatoid_Arthritis

Suggested Readings

Baird CL, Sands L. A pilot study of the effectiveness of guided imagery with progressive muscle relaxation to reduce chronic pain and mobility difficulties of osteoarthritis. *Pain Manag Nurs.* 2004;5(3):97-104.

Dominick KL, Ahern FM, Gold C, Heller DA. Health-related quality of life and health service use among older adults with osteoarthritis. *Arthritis Rheumat.* 2004;(3):326-331.

Ignatavicius D, Workman ML. *Medical-Surgical Nursing: Patient-centered Collaborative Care.* 7th ed. St. Louis, MO: Elsevier; 2013.

Kamienski M, Tate D, Vega M. The silent thief: diagnosis and management of osteoporosis. *Natl Assoc Orthopaed Nurs.* 2011;30(3):162-171.

Neill J, Belan K, Ried K. Effectiveness of non-pharmacological interventions for fatigue in adults with multiple sclerosis, rheumatoid arthritis, or systemic lupus erythematosus: a systemic review. *J Adv Nurs.* 2006;56(6):617-635.

Risley S, Thomas MA, Bray V. Rheumatoid arthritis, new standards of care: nursing implications of infliximab. *J Orthopaed Nurs.* 2004;41(8):41-49.

Rousch K. Prevention and treatment of osteoporosis in postmenopausal women: a review. *Am J Nurs.* 2011;111(8):26-35.

Zhang Y, Li X, Wang D, Guo X. Evaluation of educational program on osteoporosis awareness and prevention among nurse students in China. *Nurs Health Sci.* 2012; 14:74-80.

WHO Scientific Group on the Assessment of Osteoporosis at Primary Health Care Level. Summary Meeting Report, Brussels, Belgium, May 5-7, 2004. www.who.int/chp/topics/Osteoporosis.pdf.

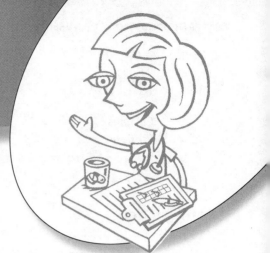

Integumentary System

LEARNING OBJECTIVES

At the end of this chapter, the reader/student will be able to:

- Discuss the anatomy and physiology of the integumentary system
- Describe common dermatologic disorders of the skin: cellulitis, psoriasis, scleroderma, and burns
- Compare treatments and nursing care for selected common skin disorders

KEY WORDS

Cellulitis   Scleroderma
Psoriasis   Burns

Introduction

The skin is composed of three layers: the epidermis, the dermis, and the sub-cutaneous tissue. New cells are formed on an ongoing basis. The epidermis is the outermost layer and the primary cell is the keratinocyte or squamous cell. Keratinocytes produce keratin, which is a resilient fibrous protein that is responsible for the vital barrier function of the skin and protects tissue from the outer environment. The dermis of second layer is beneath the epidermis and is thicker than the epidermis and provides structural support and mass to the skin. The dermis consists of connective tissue, collagen, and elastin. The third layer, the subcutaneous tissue, consists of fat cells separated by the fibrous walls of collagen and blood vessels. This layer provides a cushioning effect and anchors the other two layers to support muscle, tendons, and bone. Intact skin is the first line of defense against bacteria, foreign substances, slight trauma, heat, or ultraviolet rays. There are changes in skin as people age. The skin loses its elasticity and the skin becomes thinner, drier, and more fragile. Hair growth on the skin and the pattern indicates the person's state of health, and loss of hair or excessive hair growth can be caused by age or hormonal imbalance, thyroid disorder or ill health, or infections. There can be disorders of the skin, and some are temporary discomforts and others are chronic.

Cellulitis

A diffuse spreading of infection of the dermis and subcutaneous tissue usually on the leg and commonly due to a gram-positive bacteria and usually group A β-hemolytic streptococci. Cellulitis can occur in the orbital area, arm, pinna of the ear, or anywhere on the body. The most susceptible populations are patients with diabetes, cirrhosis, renal failure, and malnourishment; immune-compromised patients; cancer patients; and those who abuse drug and alcohol. Cellulitis typically occurs near a surgical wound, insect bites, burns, abrasions,

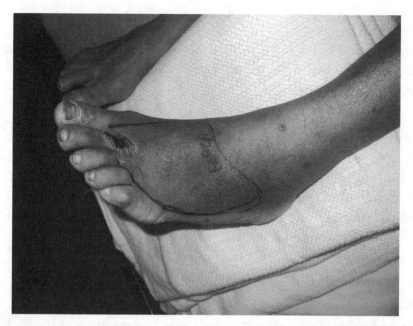

FIGURE 8–1 • Cellulitis of the foot of a diabetic person in which there is possible necrosis and gangrene of the second toe, requiring hospitalization and a podiatry consult. (Reproduced with permission from Usatine RP, et al. *The Color Atlas of Family Medicine.* New York: McGraw-Hill; 2009, figure 114-3. Courtesy of Richard P. Usatine, MD.)

lacerations, or ulcers. It usually begins as a small patch that is tender. Swelling, erythema, and pain are often present and the lesions expand over hours and the patient becomes more ill. There is also lymphadenopathy. Athlete's foot can commonly lead to cellulitis.

In small children, it is more common in the perianal region or the eye. During the acute phase of cellulitis, patients may find it too painful or sensitive to tolerate dressings or bandages. Erysipelas is a form of localized cellulitis again caused by hemolytic streptococci and *Staphylococcus aureus*. Older adults with poor host resistance are at risk for this infection. It may develop after a puncture wound, ulcer, or chronic dermatitis and can occur on the face. Before the development of antibiotics, this was a serious infection. Good hydration is important for recovery to help skin maintain its elasticity (Figure 8–1).

Clinical Manifestations

Localized pain and tenderness; erythema; fever; chills; malaise; and regional lymphadenopathy on the face, periorbital region, and neck or extremities. If eye is involved, decreased visual acuity can be symptomatic. Vesicles, blisters, hemorrhage, necrosis, or abscess may occur.

Diagnostic Tests

Complete blood count (CBC) with differential will show mild leukocytosis with a left shift early in the course. Blood cultures may be positive, and skin biopsy can be diagnostic.

Treatment

Pain can be relieved by application of Burow solution compresses. Elevation of the leg or extremity hastens recovery. Treatment with antibiotics such as penicillin, dicloxacillin, ampicillin, cephalosporin, or erythromycin is advised. Parenteral therapy is indicated for severely ill patients. Surgical debridement may be necessary if gas or purulent matter collects at site.

Nursing Interventions and Complications

Nurses must keep a detailed record of the findings with patients with cellulitis. The acronym HAMMER should be used, which represents *h*ydrate, *a*nalgesia, monitor pyrexia, *m*ark off affected, *m*easure the circumference, *e*levate, and *r*ecord. Health care professionals will be able to identify rapidly with this assessment of any signs of deterioration. Nurses should teach the family to watch for signs of impending problems. Encourage good handwashing in family. While the patient is in the hospital, nurses keep the skin moist with natural emollients and treat the patient with antibiotics and keep the patient free from any other infection.

> **CLINICAL ALERT**
>
> *Cellulitis can cause severe infection with deeper rapidly spreading infection, tissue necrosis, and severe pain. There can be marked systemic toxicity with worsening symptoms and toxic shock. If there is cellulitis of the head and neck, intubation or tracheotomy may be indicated. Nurses must monitor patients with cellulitis for any of the potential complications.*

Psoriasis

Psoriasis is a common benign, chronic inflammatory skin disease with a genetic basis. About 20%–30% have a first-degree relative with the disease. It is caused by a T-cell immunologic disorder of the skin leading to an epidermal proliferative rash characterized by well-defined brick-red papulosquamous plaques with a silvery scale.

Favored sites are the scalp, elbows, knees, palms, soles, and nails. The glans penis and vulva may be affected. Fine stippling (pitting) of the nails is highly suggestive of psoriasis. Men and women are equally affected. The extent and severity of the disease may vary widely. The first episode may be stimulated by a streptococcal pharyngitis as a child, or localized trauma. The condition is worse in the dry winter weather.

Factors that may make psoriasis worse are stress, either physical or emotional; withdrawal from steroids; folate or vitamin deficiency; alcohol use; smoking; certain drugs such as lithium, beta blockers, antimalarials, and systemic steroids. Psoriatic arthritis (rheumatoid factor negative) occurs in 5%–8% of the population with psoriasis.

Psoriasis is a chronic disorder and the course is unpredictable. Psoriasis can have a profound effect on an individual's self-image, self-esteem, and sense of well-being and can have a negative effect on all aspects of life. Psoriatic patients are at an increased risk for metabolic syndrome and lymphoma (Figure 8–2).

Clinical Manifestations

Red plaques on the affected areas may include multiple sites of scaly patches. Itching may occur, which can be very severe. Joint pain is present with psoriatic arthritis. Nails are pitted. Plaque psoriasis is deep red and begins as scaling papules that coalesce to form round-to-oval plaques and become red and inflamed. The scale may become extremely dense, especially on the scalp.

Diagnostic Tests

History and physical findings, negative rheumatoid factor, increased erythrocyte sedimentation rate, and elevated C-reactive protein may confirm diagnosis.

Treatment

For mild disease, emollient creams or topical corticosteroids; for scalp, strong-potency corticosteroid; and for moderate to severe disease, combination therapy may be used with ultraviolet light therapy as sunlight improves symptoms, and drugs such as methotrexate that block DNA synthesis in rapidly dividing epithelial cells and depresses T cells. Use of drugs such as Enbrel blocks the tumor necrosis factor. All the medications to treat psoriasis have side effects and must be monitored with labs frequently. Topical

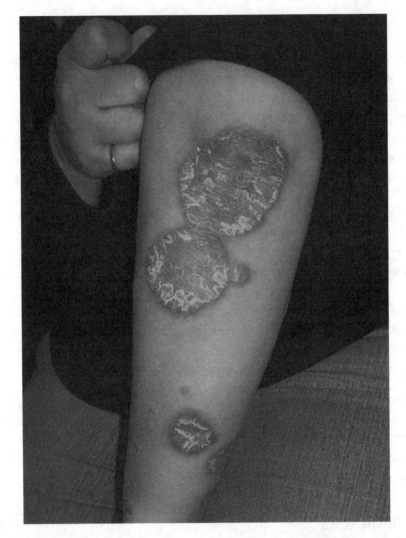

FIGURE 8–2 • Typical plaque psoriasis on the elbow and arm. (Reproduced with permission from Usatine RP, et al. *The Color Atlas of Family Medicine*. New York: McGraw-Hill; 2009, figure 145-1. Courtesy of Richard P. Usatine, MD.)

treatment is used in the vast majority of cases as 80%–90% of patients have mild to moderate psoriasis.

Nursing Interventions and Complications

Nurses play an important role in teaching and encouraging self-care of patients with skin conditions. Nurses are integral in enabling patients and their carers to make appropriate choices about their health care and to understand and make best use of available information. Nurses spend more time with patients than any other discipline.

Nurses educate patients about medication and for patients with psoriasis, continued use of their prescribed medications will decrease symptoms. Nurses also teach patients how to decrease stress utilizing strategies such as imagery as they know that stress can exacerbate symptoms.

CLINICAL ALERT

Generalized pustular psoriasis is when sterile pustules are localized or generalized and is a serious disease. Erythrodermic psoriasis in which redness is over the entire body is also a serious disease. The psychological effects of psoriasis must be evaluated, as suicide risk with chronic skin disease is a potential risk.

Scleroderma

Scleroderma is also called systemic sclerosis. It is a rare disorder characterized by diffuse fibrosis of the skin and internal organs. Symptoms usually appear during the ages 30–50s. This disease is a complex autoimmune disease. It is a multisystem connective tissue disorder that can attack a number of organ systems, including the skin, kidney, lungs, heart, and the gastrointestinal system. Deposits of excess collagen in joints, tendons, and vessels causes further damage. There are two types of scleroderma, one called limited cutaneous systemic sclerosis (lcSS) has skin involvement of the face and extremities, whereas diffuse cutaneous systemic sclerosis (dcSSc) is more extensive, with proximal skin involvement, including the chest and abdomen. The dcSS has earlier and more extensive internal organ manifestations and greater mortality. Raynaud phenomenon is usually the initial manifestation and precedes other signs by years. Raynaud is a primary vasospastic disease of the small arteries and arterioles that attacks with varying intensity and frequently affects the digits in the hand, which changes in color from white to red and feels painful in response to cold. Polyarthralgia, weight loss, and malaise are common early symptoms of diffuse scleroderma. Scleroderma is a disease that can cause ulceration in the fingertips and dysphagia due to esophageal dysfunction, and later fibrosis and atrophy of the gastrointestinal can occur. The fibrosis can also attack the pulmonary system, causing pulmonary hypertension that leads to right-sided heart failure. If renal crisis occurs, there is usually a poor outcome. This is a very distressing

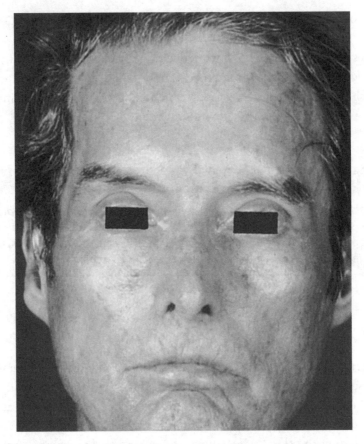

FIGURE 8–3 • Scleroderma characterized by typical expressionless, mask-like facies. (Reproduced with permission from Kasper DL, Braunwald E, Fauci AS, Hauser SL, Longo DL, Jameson JL. *Harrison's Principles of Internal Medicine*. 18th ed. New York: McGraw-Hill; 2011, figure e16-62.)

disorder that impacts physical functioning, employment, and sexuality and cause psychological distress (Figures 8–3 and 8–4).

Clinical Manifestations

Elevated blood pressure (BP)

Skin

- Digital ulceration
- Tightness and swelling of digits
- Pruritis
- Scaling of skin
- Subcutaneous calcinosis (abnormal deposits of calcium)

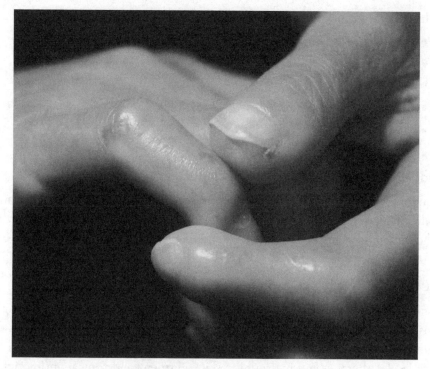

FIGURE 8–4 • Scleroderma showing sclerodactyly with tight shiny skin over the fingers. (Reproduced with permission from Usatine RP, et al. *The Color Atlas of Family Medicine*. New York: McGraw-Hill; 2009, figure 175-4. Courtesy of Everett Allen, MD.)

Joints, tendons, and bone
- Flexion contractures
- Hand swelling
- Joint stiffness
- Polyarthralgia

Gastrointestinal tract
- Dysphagia
- Esophageal reflux
- Malabsorptive diarrhea
- Weight loss
- Xerostomia (dry mouth)

Kidney
- Hypertension
- Acute renal failure

Pulmonary system

- Dry crackles at lung bases
- Dyspnea

Cardiac system

- Conduction abnormalities
- Cardiomyopathy

Diagnostic Tests

Nail fold microscopy; CBC (mild anemia); creatinine; urinalysis; antinuclear anti-bodies (ANAs); Sci-70 (systemic disease); electrocardiograph (ECG); cardiac echo; pulmonary function tests (PFTs) should be used to confirm a diagnosis.

Treatment

Treatment is symptomatic and supportive on the organ system involved: angio-tensin-converting enzyme (ACE) to preserve renal blood flow; NSAIDs for joint pain; antibiotics for secondary infections; antacids for reflux; aspirin for antiplatelet therapy; and hydrophilic skin ointment and topical antibiotics to prevent infectious cutaneous ulcers.

Nursing Interventions and Complications

Nurses must assess every system when working with scleroderma patients who have systemic disease. Assessment of the musculoskeletal, gastrointestinal, pulmonary, cardiac, and renal systems are most important. Provide psychological support for the disfigurement of face and alteration in body image. Monitor lab values, intake and output, and treat for symptoms. If the patient is in renal crisis or failure, support the patient and family and provide palliative care and end-of-life care if no further treatment is possible.

CLINICAL ALERT

The continued systemic fibrosis that occurs with scleroderma can cause death when the pulmonary system is involved. Malignant hypertension and progressive renal insufficiency occurs. If scleroderma renal crisis is not recognized early, progression to irreversible renal failure and death results. Nurses must monitor blood pressure and renal function and intervene rapidly.

Burns

Burns, also referred to as thermal injuries, occur in more than 2 million Americans each year. All age groups are affected as well as both genders. Thermal injuries affect not only the skin and its three main layers but also multiple systems. Burns are classified as superficial partial-thickness, deep partial-thickness, and full-thickness burns.

The integumentary system is obviously the most affected organ after a burn injury. Further, burns are unexpected injuries causing mental anguish aside from physical pain. After a burn injury, the catalyst of effects begins their onslaught of the body. The skin as a protective barrier, a body temperature regulator, and an indicator of nutrition and metabolic health is impaired.

Major fluid shifts occur within the first few hours (post burn phase 24–48 hours, causing hypovolemic shock). This massive fluid shift occurs because of increased capillary permeability. Loss of colloid pressures and protein potentiates this fluid shift. Life-threatening hyperkalemia can cause dysrhythmias. And in remembering that where salt goes water follows, during the acute burn phase, edema is produced. Because of the compensatory responses of the body, catecholamines are activated, causing a rise in heart rate and vasoconstriction in attempts to prevent fluid loss.

Inhalation injuries caused by facial and torso burns threaten the airway. Gases irritate the airway, causing inflammation and edema. The trachea and larynx as well as all areas of the respiratory tract are affected. The edema produces obstruction because of the inflamed tissues. Further, aspiration risks increase. The end results are hypoxia and altered pulmonary circulation. Prompt assessment that includes singed facial and nose hairs, facial burns, hoarse/brassy voice, and assessment of the mechanism of injury: fires that occurred in small tight spaces are important.

Metabolic rates rise dramatically with burn injuries. Stress hormones are excreted in response to the activation of the sympathetic nervous system. Protein breakdown occurs from muscle wasting, causing a negative nitrogen balance. The patient loses lean muscle tissue. Nutritional support either orally or parenterally is necessary to counteract the negative nitrogen balance and support the aggressive response to stress as the body attempts to heal itself.

Gastrointestinal stressors are also noted with burn injuries. Ulcerations along the mucosal area can occur especially with torso burns. Decreased circulation leads to the shedding of the mucosal lining. As the lining sloughs off, ulcerations develop. The most common type of burn-related ulcer is a Curling ulcer. The use of proton pump inhibitors (PPIs) and antacids helps reduce the incidence of burn-related ulcerations (Table 8–1).

TABLE 8–1   Guidelines for Referral to a Burn Center
Partial-thickness burns greater than 10% TBSA
Burns involving the face, hands, feet, genitalia, perineum, or major joints
Third-degree burns in any age group
Electrical burns, including lightning injury
Chemical burns
Inhalation injury
Burn injury in patients with complicated pre-existing medical disorders
Patients with burns and concomitant trauma in which the burn is the greatest risk. If the trauma is the greater immediate risk, the patient may be stabilized in a trauma center before transfer to a burn center.
Burned children in hospitals without qualified personnel for the care of children
Burn injury in patients who will require special social, emotional, or rehabilitative intervention

TBSA, total body surface area.
Reproduced with permission from Brunicardi F, et al. *Schwartz's Principles of Surgery*. 9th ed. New York: McGraw-Hill; 2009, table 8-1.

Clinical Manifestations (Local Injury)

- First-degree burns: superficial local inflammation (epidermis), pain, erythema, mild edema, skin tender to touch, pink to red
- Second-degree burns: deeper, often affecting the dermis, increased pain, inflammation and blistering of the skin may develop
- Third-degree burns: all three layers are affected extending into the subcutaneous fat and larger subcutaneous vessels, are white and leathery, usually painless because nerve endings have been damaged, black, brown, yellow, white, red
- Eschar: coagulated nonviable tissue
- Chemical burns: gray, yellow, brown, black, soft to leathery eschar, blisters, painful, depressed
- Electrical burns: must have an entry and exit wound, ischemic, yellow-white, coagulated area, iceberg effect to the wound (Figure 8–5).

Clinical Manifestations (System Injury)

- Edema (mild) or anasarca (full-body edema)
- Fluid and electrolyte imbalances

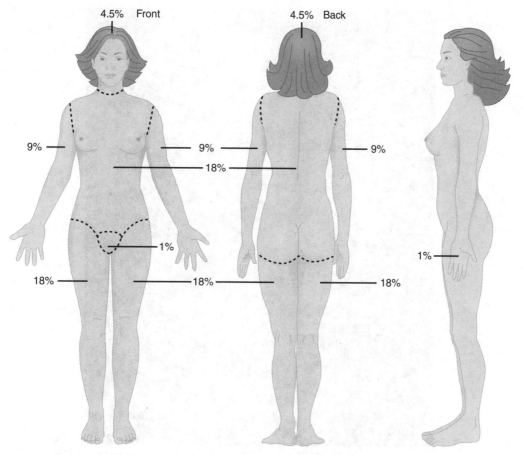

4.5% Front   4.5% Back

9%   9%   9%
18%
9%

1%

18%   18%   18%   1%

FIGURE 8–5 • The Rule of Nines can be used as a quick reference for estimating a patient's burn size by dividing the body into regions to which total body surface area is allocated in multiples of nine. (Reproduced with permission from Brunicardi F, et al. *Schwartz's Principles of Surgery*. 9th ed. New York: McGraw-Hill; 2009, figure 8-1.)

- Changes in respiratory system: laryngeal edema (stridor), aspiration, vocal cord damage (dysphonia), hypoxia, restriction of chest, development of acute respiratory distress syndrome (ARDS), development of pulmonary emboli, dyspnea, carbonaceous sputum .

- Metabolic rate: excessive stimulation of the sympathetic nervous system leads to profound excess in metabolic rate: increased body temperature, increase in respirations, heart rate, blood pressure, increases in nutritional metabolism, profound weight loss, and impaired wound healing if nutrition needs are not met (negative nitrogen balance)

- Gastric and other: development of stress ulcers, gastric necrosis, liver dysfunction, acute renal failure, skin infections (Figures 8–6 and 8–7).

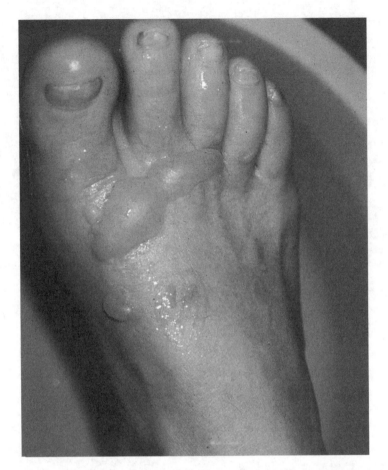

FIGURE 8–6 • Second-Degree Burn. This patient has sustained a second-degree burn to his foot. After cleansing the area, the blisters should be debrided and antimicrobial ointment should be applied. (Reproduced with permission from Knoop K, et al. *Atlas of Emergency Medicine*. 3rd ed. New York: McGraw-Hill; 2009, figure 18-43. Photo contributor: Alan B. Storrow, MD.)

Diagnostic Tests

- CT scan
- Ultrasonography
- Bronchoscopy
- Magnetic resonance imaging
- Labs: hemoglobin, hematocrit, urea nitrogen, glucose, sodium potassium, chloride, arterial blood gases (ABGs), total protein, albumin, liver function tests (LFTs), cultures: urine, sputum, blood, prothrombin time (PT), partial thromboplastin time (PTT), International Normalized Ratio (INR)

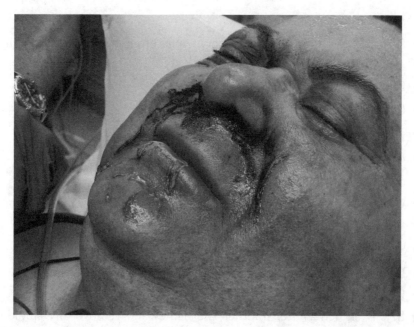

FIGURE 8–7 • Facial Burn. This patient's injury was a result of an explosion of his oxygen cannula. Ensuring that the patient has a protected airway in this type of injury is crucial. (Reproduced with permission from Knoop K, et al. *Atlas of Emergency Medicine*. 3rd ed. New York: McGraw-Hill; 2009, figure 18-44. Photo contributor: Alan B. Storrow, MD.)

Treatment

Manage airway first and a thorough examination to determine the extent of the burns and associated injuries. Large-bore intravenous (IV) access is initiated and increase fluids of Ringer lactate; insert Foley catheter for monitoring urinary output; debride burns; and thoroughly clean. Wounds that will not heal are best treated with excision and autograft. Extensive supportive care both physically and psychologically is most important in treating the burn victim.

Nursing Interventions and Complications

- Assess and support respiratory status: watch for signs and symptoms of possible airway compromise such as facial burns, singed nose hairs and eyebrows/eyelashes, brassy cough, restlessness, changes in level of consciousness, determine if burn occurred in a tight enclosed space (increases the risk of laryngeal edema and airway compromise)
- Administer oxygen therapy on an as-needed basis (PRN)

- Attain and maintain IV access
- Prepare patient for possible surgery: escharotomy (removal of the burned area of the skin)
- Pain management
- Calculate total body surface area (TBSA)
- Teach safety: smoke detector use, carbon monoxide use
- Assess airway
- Administer oxygen
- Use blanket to cover patient
- Maintain nothing-by-mouth (NPO) status
- Start IV line, infuse fluids, especially first 24 hours
- If you suspect a chemical burn, do not wet the chemicals on the skin and try to remove clothing off the patient
- If it is an active fire, smother the flames and remove any smoldering clothes
- If it is an electrical burn, move the patient from the source without jeopardizing your safety
- Start cardiac pulmonary resuscitation (CPR)
- If a radiation burn, remove clothing if possible, take patient to decontamination center, help patient shower or bathe
- Complications are airway compromise; gastrointestinal bleeding; skin infections; hypovolemia; cardiogenic shock; and sepsis

CLINICAL ALERT

The first 48 hours of burn care offers the greatest impact on morbidity and mortality of the burn victim. Nurses must be alert to the potential for abdominal compartment syndrome, which is a potentially lethal condition in severely burned patients. Markedly increased intraabdominal pressure can cause pulmonary damage and multisystem organ failure. Only 40% of patients with this complication survive. Burn patients require careful assessment and provision for optimal nutritional needs because of higher metabolism and to promote wound healing.

CASE STUDY: NURSE PRACTITIONERS

An 86-year-old white male comes to the office complaining of a rash for the last 3 days. In addition, he states he has a great deal of pain along the area of the rash and that the pain has not let him sleep. He feels tired and frustrated because he cannot understand how this rash came to be. His wife is with him and questions that he was cleaning out the backyard and although he wore long sleeves, how did he get such a rash? Both appear concerned because they have plans to visit their grandchildren the following week and might have to postpone the visit if this rash continues.

Assessment

Vesicular rash along dermal pattern on anterior and posterior aspect of the right arm.

Intense erythema noted, and visible scratch marks can be seen throughout the entire arm's length.

Upper torso assessment revealed a small patch of similar dermatologic presentation on the right scapula. Rash was not present anywhere else on the torso, posterior or anterior, abdominal area, or left arm. Nor did it cross the patient's anatomic midline. Lower extremities were free of rash as well.

Patient states that the pain felt is 9/10 on a pain scale.
BP (blood pressure): 120/82
HR (heart rate): 96
RR (respiration rate): 21
Temperature: 98.6°F
Primary malignant hypertension (PMH): hypertension, diabetes type 2
Medicines: Metformin 500 mg PO (BID), lisinopril 10 mg PO (QD)

QUESTIONS

1. What is the primary diagnosis?
2. What is (are) the various differential diagnosis?
3. What is the treatment plan? Does it involve oral, topical medications?
4. What is the follow-up plan for this patient?
5. What are the important patient teaching points for this patient and his spouse?

Suggested Readings

Amin K, Clark A, Sivakmar A, Puri A, Fox A, Brough V, Denton EM, Butler MD. The psychological impact of facial changes in scleroderma. *Psychol Health Med.* 2011;16(3):304-312.

Corall AH, Mulby AG. *Primary Care Medicine.* 4th ed. Philadelphia, PA: Lippincott Williams & Wilkins; 2000.

Domino F. *The 5 Minute Clinical Consults 2011.* 19th ed. Philadelphia, PA: Wolters Kluwer/Lippincott Williams & Wilkins; 2010.

Goroll AH, Mulley AG. *Primary Care Medicine.* 4th ed. Philadelphia, PA: Lippincott Williams & Wilkins; 2000.

Guyton AC, Hall JE. *Textbook of Medical Physiology.* 9th ed. Philadelphia, PA: W.B. Saunders; 1996.

Habif T. *Skin Disease Diagnosis and Treatment.* St. Louis, MO: Mosby; 2001.

Kelley WN. *Textbook of Internal Medicine.* 3rd ed. Philadelphia, PA: Lippincott-Raven; 1992.

Lindus L. Cellulitis. *Nurs Standard.* 2012;26(28):59.

Maguire S. Treating psoriasis in community practice. *J Community Nurs.* 2012;26(3):13-15.

McPhee SJ, Papadakis MA, Rabow MW. *2011 Current Medical Diagnosis & Treatment.* New York: McGraw-Hill; 2011.

Phipps WJ, Monhahan FD, Sands JK, Marek JF, Neighbors M. *Medical-Surgical Nursing Health and Illness Perspectives.* 7th ed. St. Louis, MO: Mosby; 2003.

Star W, Lommel LL, Shannon MT. *Women's Primary Health Care Protocols for Practice.* 2nd ed. San Francisco, CA: UCSF Nursing Press; 2004.

Taber's Cyclopedic Medical Dictionary. Philadelphia, PA: F.A. Davis; 2009.

Watkins J. Differentiating common bacterial skin infections. *Br J School Nurs.* 2012;7(2):77-78.

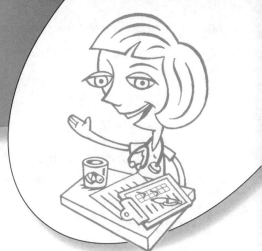

chapter 9

Sensory System

LEARNING OBJECTIVES

At the end of this chapter, the reader/student will be able to:

● Describe the physiology of the visual and auditory systems

● Compare the pathophysiology of cataracts, glaucoma, macular degeneration, and otitis media and externa, and Ménière disease

● Discuss nursing interventions/management of sensory disorders

● Monitor for complications

KEY WORDS

Cataracts	Ears
Glaucoma	Otitis Externa
Macular Degeneration	Ménière Disease

Introduction

The senses are the windows to the world. Vision and hearing are the two primary senses. The eye structure consists of accessory structures that are made of the eyelids, eyelashes, lacrimal glands, and eye muscles. These eyelids shade the eyes from light, protect the eye during sleep, and lubricate the eye to facilitate movement and visual acuity. Eyelids consist of epidermis, dermis, subcutaneous tissue, fibers of the orbicularis oculi muscle, a tarsal plate (thick connective tissue that gives the eyelids its shape), tarsal glands, and a conjunctiva. Within the tarsal plates are sebaceous glands (Meibomian glands) that secrete an oily substance. The conjunctiva is the inner portion of the eyelid.

The eyelashes protect the eye from sunlight, from foreign objects, and perspiration. Embedded with the eyelashes are sebaceous ciliary glands (glands of Zeis) that secrete lubricating fluids.

The lacrimal glands consist of excretory lacrimal ducts, lacrimal puncta, lacrimal canals, and nasolacrimal ducts. All produce and move tears (consists of salts, mucus, and lysozyme [a bactericidal enzyme]).

Eye muscles are innervated by cranial nerves III, IV, and VI. Each muscle is responsible for extrinsic eye movements to include lateral, medial, superior, and inferior movements.

Similar to the layers of the heart, the eye ball has its own set of layers: the fibrous tunic, the vascular tunic, and the retina (nervous tunic). The fibrous tunic makes up the cornea, which is a nonvascular, transparent layer that covers the colored portion of the eye, the iris. The sclera also is a portion of this tunic and it consists of a dense connective tissue that stretches over the eyeball. Between the sclera and the cornea is a juncture called the canal of Schlemm or the scleral venous sinus. The vascular tunic is the middle section. Within this section there is the choroid, the ciliary body, and the iris. Unlike the fibrous tunic, this section is highly vascularized. The choroid lines the back portion of the eye, giving it the dark color seen on fundus exams. The ciliary body is the thickest portion of the vascular tunic, and its main role is to house and move aqueous humor. Malfunction of this area causes entrapment of fluid, raising eye pressures. The iris consists of circular and radial smooth muscle fibers and is flat in nature. Within its center is the pupil. The iris and the pupil are mainly responsible for the regulation of light entering the eye. The parasympathetic and sympathetic systems regulate the opening and closing of the pupil. Both types of responses are visceral reflexes.

Finally, the retina (nervous tunic) is the third and innermost portion of the eyeball. Within the retina is the optic disc that allows the passage of blood vessels, aqueous humor, and nerves from the eyeball to the brain. The main nerve is the optic nerve. Important blood vessels include the central retinal artery and the central retinal vein. The retina also houses the most important visual sensory component: the neural portion. It is through this complex system that the brain acknowledges what the eye sees. The three layers of the neural portion noted as the eye perceives the vision, which are as follows: the photoreceptor layer (gives the person the ability to discriminate between black and white vision at night [rods] and color [cones]), the bipolar cell layers (modify and adjust visual signals for the brain to process them), and the ganglion cell layer (continued refined pathway).

Cataracts

As the population is aging and living longer, sensory problems concerning the eyes are becoming more prevalent. One of the most common optical changes among the elderly is the development of cataracts. These changes to vision as a whole contribute to risk for injury, self-care deficit disorders, and alterations in activities of daily living. However, it is important to also keep in mind that cataract formation is not exclusive to the aging population. Various reasons other than aging contribute to cataract formation. Secondary cataracts are formed in the presence of chronic diseases such as diabetes mellitus or in increased intraocular pressures (glaucoma) or with the overuse of steroids. Traumatic cataracts form secondary to blunt injury to the eyes, and in many cases the cataract may not be evident until years after the injury. Exposure to alkaline chemicals may also contribute to traumatic cataracts. Congenital cataracts are dominant gene inherited and require no intervention unless vision is impaired. The opaque lens is replaced with a synthetic lens, improving vision considerably. Finally, radiation-induced cataracts may form because of excess exposure to ultraviolet rays or other sources of radiation.

The opacity noted in cataracts is created from an inflammatory response. The cells within the eyes begin changing in response to either aging, trauma, genetics, or metabolic disease. During the degeneration process of ocular cells, water content within the cells increases. Progressive cellular destruction occurs involving the entire lens. Because the high volume of water and cellular debris cannot be contained in a small space, it leaks out into the aqueous humor of the eye. Macrophages complete the phagocytic cycle, further clouding the lens producing the cataract.

Clinical Manifestations

Most patients will begin reporting changes in their vision and visual acuity.

- Decreased ability to see in low light
- Presentation of halos
- Changes to the visual field
- Increasing intraocular pressures
- Decreased light transmission
- Changes in visual acuity
- Diplopia

Diagnostic Tests

Diagnostic tests are performed by opticians or ophthalmologists. Basic visual acuity testing is provided by most other health care professionals, including the registered nurse.

- Slit lamp or ophthalmoscope: demonstrating a loss of the normal expected red reflex behind the back of the eye
- Ultrasonography of the eye that assesses for increased opacity
- Contrast sensitivity: detects light transmission
- Pupil dilation: assess microvascular, red reflex, optic nerve, and fovea of the eye

Nursing Interventions and Complications

Aimed at protecting sensory function and at patient safety, the nurse is instrumental in teaching the patient how to manage cataracts before and after possible cataract extraction surgery.

- Assess visual acuity
- Protection of the eye: use of sunglasses in ultraviolet light, reducing risk of splashing chemicals in the eye, and a safe home environment are key for overall eye protection
- Teaching the use of proper medication instillation, especially in the presence of glaucoma, as well as side effects, adverse effects, and the therapeutic effects of eye medications.
- Monitoring metabolic diseases such as diabetes mellitus to protect from microvascular destruction
- Preoperative care: usually outpatient surgery, need for blood work, routine electrocardiography (ECG), coagulation studies, procedure, activities after procedure, turning and repositioning, administration of preoperative medications, answer patient's and family's questions regarding procedure, comprehensive physical assessment
- Postoperative care: assess intravenous fluids, vital signs, use of special eye bandages, provide emotional support, administer antibiotics if ordered, and orient patient. After cataract extraction surgery: no heavy lifting, wearing eye patch until first follow-up visit, no driving, no strenuous activities, teach patient not to rub the eye, to apply compresses as needed (warm or cool), avoidance of any activity that increases intraocular pressures: coughing, bending, jerky head movements, being constipated
- Avoid smoking
- Do not sit in direct sunlight
- Importance of follow-up appointments
- Encourage verbalization of feelings

Complications of cataracts are safety-related sensory changes, progression of a metabolic disorder, and gross activity limitations.

- Increased intraocular pressures
- Loss of sight (blind)
- Severe vision loss (significant loss but with some vision)
- Eye infections
- Falls/injury

Glaucoma

Water needs to move in order to be effective and not cause ocular damage. Within the structures of the eyes, there are numerous sites where aqueous humor is allowed to drain in appropriate amounts. At times, changes within these trabecular structures or other draining/fluid retention or functional problems occur with the eye that prevents this fluid to move freely. When this occurs, fluid builds up. As this fluid increases, it exerts pressure within the eye. This increased pressure is known as intraocular pressures.

The normal pathway for aqueous humor to flow is from the posterior portion of the eye to the eye's anterior chamber via the pupil. Through the trabecular mesh of the intricate eye structures, the fluid is drained into venous circulation through specialized pathways known as the canal of Schlemm. The intraocular pressures that are generally measured are indicative of the balance between production of fluid and absorption of aqueous humor. Normal intraocular pressures range between 10 and 21 mm Hg.

There are two basic forms of glaucoma: open-angle glaucoma and closed-angle (narrow-angle) glaucoma. Of the two, the most dangerous one is closed angle because if left untreated, will cause loss of vision fairly rapidly. In open-angle glaucoma, the anterior chamber is open and able to release the flow of fluid but something is obstructing via the trabecular mesh of the eye. In closed-angle glaucoma, the anterior chamber is closed, thus not allowing the fluid to exit via the canal of Schlemm. Rapid buildup of pressures occurs denoting the danger in high pressures and loss of vision (Figure 9–1).

Clinical Manifestations

As with most visual problems, changes in visual acuity are key. In glaucoma, the most significant visual disturbance is the loss of peripheral vision.

- Sometimes the visual changes are progressive and not noticeable for years
- Difficulty with vision in the dark
- Diplopia
- Problems with focusing on objects nearby
- In closed-angle glaucoma: acute sharp eye pain, cloudy vision, halos, a rigid eyeball, increased intraocular pressure, and associated constitutional symptoms of nausea and vomiting

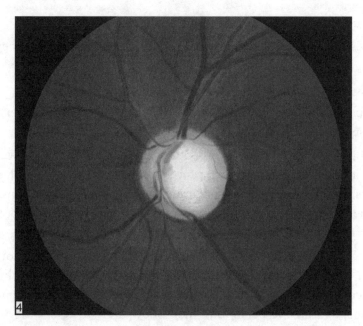

FIGURE 9–1 • A 50-year-old man with glaucoma has an increased optic cup-to-disc ratio of 0.8. Median cup-to-disc ratio is 0.2–0.3, but varies considerably among individuals. (Reproduced with permission from Usatine RP, et al. *The Color Atlas of Family Medicine*. New York: McGraw-Hill; 2009, figure 18-1. Courtesy of Paul D. Comeau, MD.)

Diagnostic Tests

Measurement of intraocular pressures is the mainstay of glaucoma as is a detailed family history because the propensity for its development has a genetic disposition.

- Tonometry: measures intraocular pressures
- Dilated fundus exam: microvascular assessment
- Peripheral field test: assessment of peripheral vision
- Gonioscopy: assessment of the anterior chamber angle
- Pachymetry: assessment and measurement of the thickness of the cornea (which can contribute to sluggish fluid movement)

Nursing Interventions and Complications

- Assessment of visual acuity
- Medication administration and application: β-adrenergic blockers, adrenergic agonists, carbonic anhydrase inhibitors, β-adrenergic blockers, prostaglandin analogs, and miotic agents to help improve the flow of fluid

- Diet: fluid and sodium restrictions
- Assessment and proper management of eye pain; monitoring for eye complications as manifested by excruciating eye pain
- Encourage verbalization of feelings
- Prepare patient for possible corrective surgery: iridotomy (laser), gonioplasty (laser), or trabecular mesh repair, trabeculectomy.
- Preoperative care: usually outpatient surgery, need for blood work, routine ECG, coagulation studies, procedure, activities after procedure, turning and repositioning, administration of preoperative medications, answer patient's and family's questions regarding procedure, comprehensive physical assessment
- Postoperative care: assess intravenous fluids, vital signs, use of special eye bandages, provide emotional support, administer antibiotics if ordered, and orient patient. After cataract extraction surgery: no heavy lifting, wearing eye patch until first follow-up visit, no driving, no strenuous activities, teach patient not to rub the eye, to apply compresses as needed (warm or cool), avoidance of any activity that increases intraocular pressures: coughing, bending, jerky head movements, or being constipated

Dependent on the type of glaucoma presentation, closed-angle glaucoma carries the greatest risk for vision loss (blindness)

- Increased intraocular pressures
- Loss of sight (blind)
- Severe vision loss (significant loss but with some vision)
- Eye infections
- Falls/injury

Macular Degeneration

The retina is the soul of the eyes. In its center is the macula. A small indentation made up of cone cells, the macula is responsible for visual acuity. In macular degeneration, destruction of the macula occurs and eventually, over time, there is a loss of vision. While the exact etiology of macular degeneration remains unknown, there is an indirect correlation with aging, smokers, being female, and being Caucasian. There is strong suspicion that there might be a genetic link to the disease as well. Unlike glaucoma where there is preservation of central vision with destruction of peripheral vision, in macular degeneration, there is loss of central vision with preservation of peripheral vision.

As the retina ages, the macula's ability to acutely return vision is diminished. Age-related macular changes involve nonneovascular changes and neovascular changes. Nonneovascular or dry (nonexudative) macular degeneration involves the development of drusens (yellowish patches) that eventually coalesce within the eye, blocking vision. The blood vessels, small capillaries that surround the macula, do not leak blood, which is the reason it is called dry or nonneovascular macular degeneration. In neovascular degeneration, within the choroid areas of the eyes (the area where a vast compilation of microvessels congregate), new vessels tend to form in response to macular changes. These newly formed vessels are weak and leak blood. These tiny hemorrhagic spots cause eventual scar tissue, with subsequent loss of vision. Changes that occur in both wet and dry are irreversible (Figure 9–2).

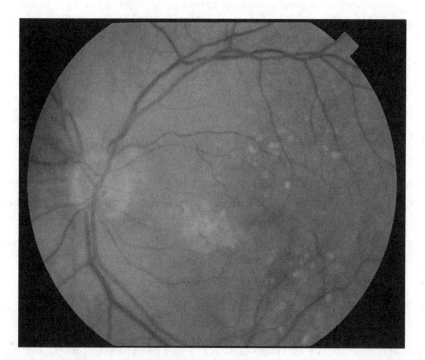

FIGURE 9–2 • Intermediate dry age-related macular degeneration with macular depigmentation and drusen (yellowish-colored subretinaldeposits on the macula). This patient has central vision distortion. (Reproduced with permission from Usatine RP, et al. *The Color Atlas of Family Medicine.* New York: McGraw-Hill; 2009, figure 22-1. Courtesy of Paul D. Comeau, MD.)

Clinical Manifestations

Nonneovascular (dry) macular degeneration:

- Gradual loss of central vision
- Inability to recognize colors
- Is painless

Neovascular (wet) macular degeneration:

- Sudden and aggressive loss of vision
- Distorted wiggly lines (metamorphopsia)
- Depth distortion

Diagnostic Tests

- Dilated pupil examination assessing for drusen formation or hemorrhages
- Amsler grid test assessing for waviness (metamorphopsia)
- Fluorescein angiogram where a dye is injected into general circulation and then assessed as it passes through the small vessels of the eyes looking for leaking blood vessels

Nursing Interventions and Complications

- Monitor visual acuity
- Prevent injury/falls
- Prepare patient for treatments: laser photocoagulation, photodynamic therapy

  Management of patient after medication therapy: protect from eye injury, falls, increase in intraocular pressures, transient visual changes, direct sunlight, increasing eye discomfort, increasing photosensitivity, infection/redness of the eyes, blurry vision, or an increase in the number of floaters within vision.

- Prompt medical follow-up after treatments
- Administration of antioxidant protection: vitamin C, zinc, β-carotene (vitamin A), vitamin E

Irreversible changes to vision that leave the patient completely unable to maintain central vision. Remembering that peripheral vision remains intact, proper and timely assessment of intraocular pressures to preserve peripheral vision is paramount.

Ears

Introduction

The ears, located laterally to the skull, have two main functions: receptors of sound waves that are translated into sound, hence hearing abilities and equilibrium. There are three main portions to the ears: the outer ear (external), the middle ear, and the inner (internal) ear. Outside the brain where the skinfolds open to the ear are portions known as the auricle. The auricle consists of two parts: the helix, which is the upper portion, and the lobule, the lower portion.

Hearing

The external ear is the first place that a sound wave encounters. The sound wave passes through the external auditory canal (meatus) into the eardrum, which vibrates as the sound wave passes through it. Compression and decompression of the air contributes to this vibration. The malleus, the first bone, also vibrates. Movement of the sound wave from the malleus extends to the incus and then to the stapes (small bones within the ears). As the third bone, the stapes, vibrates, fluid pressure changes. Pressure changes throughout the sound wave moving through the auditory system causes bulging of structures. As the pressure continues to fluctuate, additional structures within the ear respond (the vestibuli and scala tympani, the vestibular membrane, the basilar membrane, and the hair cells of the spiral organ). Hair cells move to the pressure changes, thus producing receptor potentials that generate a nerve impulse along cranial nerve (CN) VIII. Sound is perceived and interpreted.

Sound waves that are heard with human ears are measured in frequencies. The human ear can hear between 1,000 and 4,000 Hz (Hertz) per second. Sound intensity is measured in size of vibrations or decibels (dB). Loud sounds to the point of discomfort are sounds higher than 120 dB, painful at higher than 140 dB.

Equilibrium

The ability to sense position and posture is not just the role of the musculoskeletal system. The vestibular system within the ears plays a major portion on balance and movement. Two types of equilibrium exist: static equilibrium (body positioning in relation to forces of gravity) and dynamic equilibrium (body positioning in relation to movement: rotation, acceleration, and deceleration).

The vestibular system consists of vestibular branches of the CN VIII. The branches lead into hair cells (receptor cells) into the otolithic (consists of calcium carbonate crystals) membrane. All are firmly rooted within a basement membrane. Via the depolarization or hyperpolarization of hair cells, afferent and efferent nerve fibers send fast or slow impulses to the brain. When the head moves, these hairs vacillate or bend forward or backward. This motion regulates the delicate vestibular system. Increased fluid or ear effusions hamper the movement of these hairs, causing dizziness seen in vertigo states or Ménière disease.

Otitis Media

Otitis media is a bacterial infection of the ear that is centered around the temporal bone and its surrounding space. The infection can present acutely or chronically. In the presence of acute otitis media, there is often an accompanying upper respiratory tract infection. Although the infection can present at any age, infants and children are most susceptible because of their smaller Eustachian tubes.

Otitis media usually presents rapidly and can have effects lasting up to 3 weeks after initial presentation. The Eustachian tubes open and close to allow for fluid to drain and to help maintain equal pressure within the ears. Dysfunction of the tubes can cause fluid accumulation that introduces bacteria and causes infection of the mucosal lining of the middle ear to occur once it opens to accommodate for pressure changes. Infection of the mucosal lining of the middle ear will then occur.

Clinical Manifestations

- Otalgia
- Aural pressure
- Decreased/diminished hearing
- Fever
- Irritability
- Erythemic ears

Diagnostic Tests

- Otoscopic examination
- Audiometry: if hearing loss is suspected (including Whisper test, Weber test, and Rinne test)

- Tympanogram
- Auditory brainstem response test
- Electronystagmography: used to assess oculomotor and vestibular systems
- Middle ear endoscopy

Nursing Interventions and Complications

- Teach patient not to insert foreign objects into the ear (Q-tips, bobby-pins, nails, etc.)
- Avoid trauma to the ear because it can lead to infection
- Avoid getting ears wet: swimming, washing hair. A petrolatum-moistened cotton ball inserted gently into the ear canal will eliminate moist pockets that can lead to infection
- Use of otic drops after swimming that dry up the ear canal
- Assessment of chronic ear infections
- Assess hearing acuity
- Use of otic and/or systemic antibiotics
- Prepare patient for possible surgery: tympanoplasty, ossiculoplasty, mastoidectomy, myringotomy—infection prevention, verbalization of fears/anxiety, medication administration, improving communication, self-care, prevent falls/injury, assess sensory perception, assess for risk of isolation, assess for body image disturbance
- Mastoiditis: fever, jaw pain. Usually seen weeks after undertreated or inadequately treated acute otitis media
- Petrous apicitis: palsy of CN VI, purulent drainage, deep ear pain
- Central nervous system (CNS) infection: meningitis
- Facial paralysis: seen with either acute/chronic otitis media, CN VII inflammation
- Sigmoid sinus thrombosis: infection of the sinus that leads to septicemia

Otitis Externa

Otitis externa is often present in situations where moisture has been trapped within the inner ear, setting the stage for the growth of bacteria. The bugs of choice include *Pseudomonas*, *Proteus*, or *Aspergillus*.

Inflammation and/or infection of the external aspect of the ear can range from mild to severe. The severity of the inflammation/infection can cause cellulitis and abscesses. Commonly seen in the summer secondary to water in the ears after swimming, it can cause severe pain and discomfort. Inflammation of the pinna can be also quite painful on manipulation of the ear. If cellulitis of the auricle and external auditory canal is present, the patient may complain of acute symptoms.

Clinical Manifestations

- Otalgia
- Pruritus
- Purulent drainage
- Fever
- Erythema
- Firmness along pinna
- Itching

Diagnostic Tests

- Otoscopic examination
- Audiometry: if hearing loss is suspected (including Whisper test, Weber test, and Rinne test)
- Tympanogram
- Auditory brainstem response test
- Electronystagmography: used to assess oculomotor and vestibular systems
- Middle ear endoscopy

Nursing Interventions and Complications

- Teach patient not to insert foreign objects into the ear (Q-tips, bobby-pins, nails, etc.)
- Avoid trauma to the ear because it can lead to infection
- Avoid getting ears wet: swimming, washing hair. A petrolatum-moistened cotton ball inserted gently into the ear canal will eliminate moist pockets that can lead to infection

- Use of otic drops after swimming that dry up the ear canal
- Assessment of chronic ear infections
- Assess hearing acuity
- Administration of analgesics
- Administration of otic medication either by dropper or by using a wick into the inner ear when it is edematous and otic antibiotics are needed
- Malignant external otitis infection: persistent otitis infection especially seen in diabetic patients, cancer patients, and others who are immuno-compromised. Osteomyelitis develops on the floor of the ear canal and extends inward. Progressive cranial nerve involvement ensues: CN VI, VII, IX, X, XI and/or XII

Ménière Disease

Also known as endolymphatic hydrops, Ménière disease involves an inner ear imbalance of the vestibular system of the ears.

Etiology is unknown but there is suspicion that head trauma or exposure to syphilis may have an indirect link to its presentation.

Within the inner ear, there is an area known as the endolymphatic compartment. Within this compartment lies a membranous endolymphatic sac that lies between the temporal bone and partly within the dura of the posterior fossa. Through this compartment, a fluid called endolymph flows through. This intracellular fluid contains large amounts of potassium and small amounts of sodium. When this compartment becomes distended, changes in pressure develop, causing hearing loss, vertigo, and tinnitus. The mechanisms that potentiate the development of Ménière disease are largely unknown, but some clinical situations may cause its development. They include trauma to the ear, acute/chronic ear infections, immunologic imbalances, endocrinologic problems such as problems with the adrenal glands, or with the thyroid. Hearing loss is progressive and initially unilateral. As time goes by, the hearing loss is bilateral and the patient becomes deaf. The primary disability for this patient is acute irreversible hearing loss.

Clinical Manifestations

One of the important things to keep in mind with clinical manifestations of Ménière disease is that many times the symptoms wax and wane. There may or may not be episodes of associated migraine-type headaches along with the classical symptoms.

- Episodic vertigo
- Decreased/diminished hearing loss
- Tinnitus
- Aural pressure
- Nausea/vomiting
- Dizziness

Diagnostic Tests

- Platform posturography: done in the presence of vertigo
- Sinusoidal harmonic acceleration test
- Middle-ear endoscopy
- Audiometry
- Weber test

Nursing Interventions and Complications

- Assessment of hearing acuity
- Administration of medications: meclizine HCl (Antivert), diazepam (Valium), promethazine HCl (Phenergan), or diuretics
- Teach dietary: low sodium, maintaining hydration, avoidance of caffeine, limit or stop alcohol consumption, avoid monosodium glutamate (MSG), avoiding any medications that contain aspirin.
- Prepare patient for surgery: endolymphatic sac decompression or vestibular nerve sectioning infection prevention, verbalization of fears/anxiety, medication administration, improving communication, self-care, prevent falls/injury, assess sensory perception, assess for risk of isolation, assess for body image disturbance
- Maintain patient safety
- Progressive hearing loss
- Risk for falls due to sensory deprivation
- Depression/anxiety
- Social isolation

REVIEW QUESTIONS

1. **What important patient teaching would be necessary for a patient with sensory deficits that include increased intraocular pressure and mild hearing loss?**

    A. Instruct the patient to turn all lights in her living space to reduce the incidence of falls

    B. Instruct the patient to put her hearing aid on the loudest volume possible

    C. Instruct the patient to speak as loud as possible so she can hear herself speak and avoid communication deficits

    D. Instruct the patient to use ear plugs to listen to music so she can get the full benefit of musical therapy

2. **All of the following are expected behavioral manifestations of an elderly person that is suffering from sensory deficit except:**

    A. Depression

    B. Anxiety

    C. Anger

    D. Euphoria

Suggested Readings

Ervin SE. Meniere's disease: identifying classic symptoms and current treatments. *AAOHN J.* 2004;52(4):156-158.

Fitzgerald MA. Acute otitis media in an era of drug resistance: implications for NP practice. *Nurse Pract.* 1999;24(10):10-14.

Houde SC, Huff MH. Age-related vision loss in older adults: a challenge for gerontological nurses. *J Gerontol Nurs.* 2003;29(4):25-33.

Ignatavicius D, Workman ML. *Medical-Surgical Nursing: Patient-Centered Collaborative Care.* 7th ed. St. Louis: MO: Elsevier; 2013.

Lip PL, Menon V. Age-related macular degeneration: an overview and update. *Therapy.* 2006;3(3):417-424.

Montville NH, White MA. Diagnosis and pharmacological management of acute otitis media. *Pediatr Nurs.* 1998;24(5):423-429.

Pritchard MJ. Understanding Meniere's disease 1: causes and diagnosis. *Nurs Times.* 2007;103:28-29.

Pritchard MJ. Understanding Meniere's disease 2: treatment options. *Nurs Times.* 2007;103:30-31.

Schmier JK, Covert DW, Lau EC. Patterns and costs associated with progression of age-related macular degeneration. *Am J Ophthalmol.* 2012;154(4):675-681.e1.

Watkinson S. Management of visual impairment in older people: what can the nurse do? *Aging Health*. 2009;5(6):821-832.

Watkinson S. Visual impairment in older people. *Nurs Older People*. 2009;21(8): 30-36.

Weih LM, VanNewkirk MR, McCarty CA, Taylor HR. Age-specific causes of bilateral visual impairment. *Arch Ophthalmol*. 2000;118(2):264-269.

chapter **10**

Hematologic System

LEARNING OBJECTIVES

At the end of this chapter, the reader/student will be able to:

- Describe the physiology of anemias, leukemia, and Hodgkin disease as a collective group
- Compare the pathophysiology of: aplastic anemia, sickle cell anemia, pernicious anemia, folate deficiency and iron deficiency anemia, leukemia and Hodgkin versus non-Hodgkin lymphoma
- Discuss nursing interventions/management of all hematologic disorders
- Monitor for complications in each category

> ## KEY WORDS
>
> Aplastic Anemia
> Sickle Cell Anemia
> Folate Deficiency
> Iron Deficiency Anemia
>
> Leukemia
> Hodgkin/Non-Hodgkin Lymphoma
> Multiple Myeloma

Introduction

This is a general discussion on anemia and the various causes. Anemias can occur because of red blood cell (RBC) destruction, excessive loss of RBCs, or impaired formation of RBCs. Understanding the morphology of RBCs is important in understanding the type of anemia a patient may have. A normocytic/normochromic RBC is considered normal. The RBC size is normal and its color (iron saturation level) is normal. They are of uniform size and shape throughout. A microcytic/hypochromic RBC is a small, pale cell. These cells develop when there is an impairment in the synthesis of hemoglobin. The macrocytic cell is large and is normochromic. When cells are anisocytic, this is a collection of RBCs that together include larger and smaller ones, and usually all are normochromic. Poikilocytosis refers to particular shapes of RBCs specific to a disease. For example, in sickle cell anemia, the cell is C-shaped; in thalassemia, the cells are large, with openings in the center.

Aplastic Anemia

When the bone marrow is unable to produce sufficient RBCs, the resultant anemia is known as aplastic anemia. The stem cells from which RBCs mature are decreased in quantity and other blood-forming cells fail to mature. This type of anemia often carries a poorer prognosis and, at times, the etiology for why it presents is not understood. There is speculation that Fanconi anemia, a genetic aberrancy, may be one of the causes—or when there is overwhelming cell destruction, such as when chemotherapeutic or radiative agents are introduced into the body. Other causes may include any disease that causes immune suppression, infections (Epstein-Barr virus [EBV] or cytomegalovirus [CMV], hepatitis), vitamin B_{12} deficiency, or drugs (phenytoin, indomethacin, chemotherapeutic agents, etc.) as well as drugs that suppress the immune system in transplant patients. Drug toxicity with arsenic, insecticides, paint thinners, or benzene are other causative factors. The cells of aplastic anemia are normocytic, and normochromic in nature.

Clinical Manifestations

Symptoms are usually gradual, and patients often first present with bleeding as a low platelet count is usually present.

- Weakness
- Dyspnea
- Headache
- Syncope
- Weakness
- Petechiae
- Bleeding: gums, vagina, and gastrointestinal (GI) tract
- Infections
- Pallor
- Fatigue
- Ecchymosis

Diagnostic Tests

- Complete blood count to include platelets
- Bone marrow biopsy

Treatment

Treatments center on bone marrow replacement or blood transfusions. As with any transplant, rejection is a major consideration but fortunately only occur in a relatively small percentage of patients. Immunosuppressive modalities are alternative choices, especially for those that are not candidates for bone marrow transplantation.

Nursing Interventions and Complications

Patient should be monitored for complication closely. Because many of the reasons aplastic anemia develops are due to a compromised host, measures to anticipate complications are important. Infection control, monitoring vital signs, preparing patient for transfusions, and reducing exposure to agents that can further exacerbate the anemia should be implemented.

Sickle Cell Anemia

Sickle cell anemia (SCA) is a genetic disorder of the RBC. Sickle cell is an autosomal recessive disorder. The normal constituents of amino acid, glutamic acid, is replaced by a hemoglobin molecule called valine. Valine causes a displacement of the hemoglobin chains. The population most susceptible to this genetic disorder are the African Americans, because they tend to carry the sickle cell trait. The RBC is shaped like a C and carries a low oxygen tension. The sickle cell has a life span of 10–15 days unlike that of the normal RBC of 120 days. Most people will not be symptomatic until a crisis occurs. Crises are defined as vaso-occlusive, which is the most common; anemic crisis, where a folate deficiency develops; aplastic crisis, where there is a suppression of RBCs; acute sequestration crisis, where there is liver and spleen enlargement; and a hemolytic crisis, which is rare, but destructive. Here, infection is the causative factor. RBCs of SCA are classified as poikilocytosis.

Clinical Manifestations

Oftentimes, patients may not know they have SCA until they are in crisis. Sickle cell crisis is precipitated by a few factors. The most important one is dehydration.

- Pain
- Hepatosplenomegaly
- Jaundice
- Development of gallstones
- Organ malfunction
- Spleen infarction (due to trapped hemolyzed RBC fragments)

Diagnostic Tests

Sickle cell is diagnosed by electrophoresis of the RBC, levels of hematocrit and hemoglobin (which tend to be low), and a discernable pattern to the RBC.

Nursing Interventions and Complications

Monitoring for complications is important. Patients can hemorrhage in the brain, can develop vaso-occlusive pain that is very severe in nature, or they may develop acute chest syndrome. Common sites for the pain are the abdomen, bones/joints, and the chest. Acute chest syndrome is a form of pneumonia due to multiple pulmonary infarctions that produce pulmonary infiltrates. Monitoring the patient carefully for shortness of breath, fever, chest pain, vital sign changes, progressive airway compromise, and oxygen saturation are warranted. As pulmonary infarct can occur, so can brain infarcts. Another major complication of SCA is stroke.

Patients in sickle cell crisis require prompt intravenous (IV) hydration and pain management. Anticipating pain and considering breakthrough pain medications are important assessments of the nurse.

Finally, patients in SCA crisis are prone to infection. Because of the possible infarcts of the spleen or congestion due to hemolyzed RBCs, the spleen would be unable to provide its support in fighting infection. Severe spleen compromise puts the patient at risk for infection. Timely assessment and intervention is necessary.

Folate Deficiency

Folate can be found in many foods such as green leafy vegetables and fruits. Other food items that may contain folate are cereals. However, once the food is cooked, the benefit of folate is lost. Folate is an important catalyst for DNA synthesis and RBC formation. Deficiencies potentiate vitamin B_{12}-deficient anemia. This type of anemia is mostly found in the alcoholic whose nutrient intake is often decreased and in any other patient with a malabsorption syndrome or poor nutrition in general. Some medications that interfere with the absorption of folate in the gut include phenytoin, diuretics, and methotrexate. RBCs in folate deficiency are macrocytic.

Clinical Manifestations

- Anemia (MCV > 100 fL)
- Underlying neurological manifestations (difficulty concentrating, declining cognition, forgetfulness
- Fatigue
- Dizziness

- Irritable
- Anorexia
- Weight loss
- Weakness

Diagnostic Tests

- Complete blood count to include platelets
- Nutritional consult
- Weighing patient daily
- Albumin levels
- Vitamin B_{12} levels
- RBC indices

Treatment

- Nutritional consult
- Intake of foods high in folic acid: beef, liver, broccoli, peanut butter, red beans, oatmeal, and asparagus
- Vitamin B_{12} IM injections

Iron Deficiency Anemia

Iron deficiency anemia (IDA) is a common anemia. Found around the globe, there is a dietary indiscretion with this anemia. It can also occur because of excessive bleeding (menstruation, GI ulcers, cancer, or hemorrhoids). RBCs as such are quite efficient. At the end of their life span, their iron content is broken down and reabsorbed by newly matured RBCs. Some iron, however, is lost through feces and must be replaced by diet. With chronic blood loss, iron cannot be reabsorbed and utilized over and over.

Clinical Manifestations

Symptoms develop when extreme iron loss is evident.

- Fatigue
- Pallor
- Weakness

- Shortness of breath
- Tachycardia

Diagnostic Tests

- Complete blood count including hematocrit and hemoglobin levels
- RBC indices
- Occult blood monitoring

Treatment

- Iron supplements (ferrous sulfate)
- Nutrition 325 mg (QD) orally consult
- Monitoring use of aspirin/nonsteroidal anti-inflammatory drugs (NSAIDs) that can cause GI bleeding

Nursing Interventions and Complications

Patient education in terms of nutrition is important. Diets rich in iron should be taught to the patient. Excessive use of aspirin or NSAIDs should be monitored to prevent GI ulcers. Gastric ulcers/peptic ulcers are a major cause of iron deficiency. Complications can include occult bleeding or frank bleeding such as with hemorrhoids. Patients should report these symptoms immediately. Assist the patient with activities of daily living (ADLs) as fatigue is a constant factor. Provide frequent oral care as certain types of anemia cause a swollen tongue. Monitor vital signs closely and assess the patient for pallor, edema, or any circulatory compromise. Listen to lung and heart sounds routinely. Iron supplements may be given orally or via injection. To preserve the injected medication and to prevent skin trauma, iron injections are delivered using the Z-track method.

CLINICAL ALERT

Hemorrhage and hemorrhage complications can be significant. Patient education is the key to prevention. Appropriate dietary counseling and food preparation are important measures for good dietary intake of iron.

Leukemia

When the body's white blood cells (WBCs) go awry, leukemias are born. Leukemias are named according to the dominant WBC affected. It accounts for approximately 10% of all cancers and it does not know race, ethnicity, or gender. The aberrant WBCs begin their malignant process within the confines of the bone marrow but soon find their way into other tissues. Within the bone marrow, malignant cells proliferate and therefore prevent the bone marrow from producing healthy WBCs and RBCs. Platelet production is also affected. This in turn impairs immune function. Children often have a more promising prognosis than adults. Because the main fighting cell within the body's defenses is affected, patients succumb to infection, anemia, and thrombocytopenia.

There are four types of leukemia: chronic lymphocytic leukemia (CLL), acute lymphoblastic leukemia (ALL), chronic myeloid leukemia (CML), and acute myeloid leukemia (AML). Of these leukemias, CLL is the common form of WBC aberrancy.

Who develops this white blood aberrancy is difficult to stratify. Twins and those with Down syndrome have a 20-fold increased risk as well as those that inherit the Philadelphia chromosome. Exposure to toxins has played a role. These include arsenic, benzene, pesticides, and chemotherapeutic agents. Leukemias that develop using chemotherapeutic agents for another type of cancer are called secondary leukemias (Figures 10–1 and 10–2).

Clinical Manifestations

Symptoms are generally different between acute and chronic presentations of leukemia.

Acute
- Oral infections or thrush
- Hyperplasia of the gums and gum line
- Epistaxis
- Petechiae
- Vascular occlusions
- Chills
- Bone pain
- Joint pain

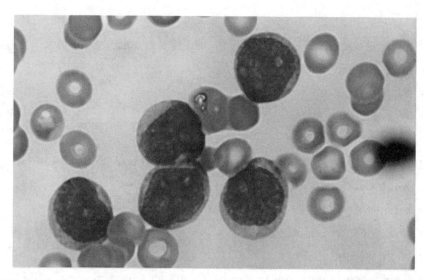

FIGURE 10–1 • Acute myelogenous leukemia, with minimal maturation. Blood film. Five leukemic myeloblasts. Each contains several nucleoli some of which are very large. High nuclear-to-cytoplasmic ratio. Agranular cytoplasm. (Reproduced with permission from Lichtman M, et al. *Williams Hematology*. 7th ed, New York: McGraw-Hill; 2005, figure VI A-1. Courtesy of Marshall Lichtman.)

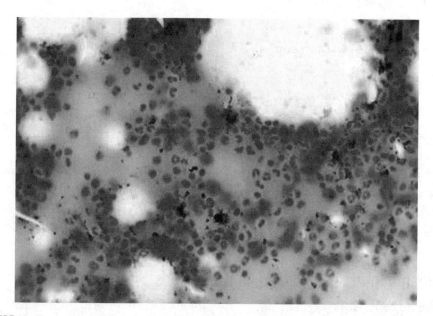

FIGURE 10–2 • Increased iron aggregates. Marrow. Prussian blue stain. Several macrophages engorged with iron are noted. The frequency of iron aggregates is greater than that seen in normal marrow. Marrow iron is contained in two proteins: hemosiderin and ferritin. Prussian blue stains hemosiderin iron, and macrophage iron is principally hemosiderin. In iron-deficient states, loss of marrow storage iron in hemosiderin and ferritin is proportionately similar, and thus staining for hemosiderin is a reasonable measure of storage iron. (Reproduced with permission from Lichtman M, et al. *Williams Hematology*. 7th ed, New York: McGraw-Hill; 2005, figure V B-1. Courtesy of Marshall Lichtman.)

Chronic

- Hypermetabolic symptoms: fever, palpitations, and weight loss
- Splenomegaly/hepatomegaly
- Diaphoresis
- Weakness
- Bone pain/tenderness
- Lymphadenopathy (chronic—scalp, pleura, GI tract, prostate, and liver)
- Anorexia
- Fatigue
- Low-grade temperatures
- Night sweats
- CNS involvement: nausea, vomiting, papilledema, and coma

Diagnostic Tests

- Complete blood count
- Microscopic analysis of blood
- Bone marrow aspiration
- Cytogenetic studies
- Computed tomographic (CT) scan: abdomen, chest, and pelvis

Treatment

For acute leukemias, the treatment of choice is chemotherapy. Chemotherapy, especially in ALL in children, yields a high remission rate. For the chronic leukemias, bone marrow transplant is a treatment that is considered in CML. Chemotherapy treatment may be also effective.

Nursing Interventions and Complications

The nurse must be vigilant in her assessment and monitoring of the patient with leukemia. Because infection is a constant threat, hand washing is paramount. So is the maintenance of an aseptic protocol. Monitoring of lines such as indwelling catheters, IV lines, central lines, and wounds are critical. The nurse should also closely monitor the oral mucosa as chemotherapy can cause stomatitis, thus causing pain and a reduction in food intake. Monitor the patient for bleeding from the gums, nose, vagina, rectum, and all intravenous lines. If the patient becomes neutropenic, institute neutropenic precautions. Facilitate communication between health care providers, the patient, and his or her family.

CLINICAL ALERT

Infection control and management are paramount. All portals of entry for infection should be monitored and interventions promptly instituted. Address any psychosocial concerns the patient may have and assist with the grieving process of acute or chronic malignancies.

Hodgkin/Non-Hodgkin Lymphoma

Malignancies that begin within the lymph tissue are called lymphomas.

Hodgkin lymphoma (HL) and non-Hodgkin lymphoma (NHL) are two distinct yet similar diseases of the lymph tissue. Hodgkin is characteristic with the presence of Reed-Sternberg (R-S) cells. These cells are malignant, arising from the lymphoid tissue. The R-S cells come in various forms: popcorn cells, lacunar cells, mummified cells, as well as the common R-S presentation of a lobular cell. Hodgkin presents in a single lymph node or a chain of lymph nodes, and this spreads contiguously. Spread of neoplastic cells is in a predictable systemic pattern. The etiology of HL is largely unknown; however, there appears to be a link with exposure to EBV. HL is classified into stages I–IV, with stage I involving one single lymph node, to stage IV, which encompasses diffuse or disseminated lymph node involvement as well as extralymphatic tissue expression of disease (bone marrow, liver, lungs).

Non-Hodgkin lymphoma (NHL) is the neoplasm of B and T cells. As with HL, the etiology is unknown but malfunctions of the immune system that allows malignant cells to proliferate without detection may be a clue, for example, the patient receiving chemotherapy or the patient with HIV/AIDS. As with HL, EBV exposure is a possibility. Unlike HL, the degree and spread of lymph node involvement is unpredictable and occurs in a haphazard pattern. NHL is staged as follows: low grade, intermediate grade, and high grade. In addition, there is a separate category for NHL that cannot be graded known as the miscellaneous category.

The World Health Organization classifies HL into two categories:

- Nodular lymphocyte-predominant Hodgkin lymphoma
- Classic lymphoma

Further, the World Health Organization also classifies non-HL into two categories:

- B-Cell lymphomas (follicular lymphoma, diffuse large C-cell lymphoma, Burkitt lymphoma, marginal zone lymphoma, and mantle cell lymphoma)
- T-Cell lymphomas

Clinical Manifestations

Hodgkin lymphoma

- Lymph node enlargement: supraclavicular, axilla, and neck
- Cough
- Chest pain
- Chest x-ray finding of a mediastinal mass
- Dyspnea
- Fever, chills
- Night sweats
- Weight loss
- Pruritis
- Fatigue
- Anemia

Non-Hodgkin lymphoma

- Painless lymphadenopathy
- Fever, chills
- Weight loss
- Night sweats
- Headaches
- Visual disturbances
- Chest pain
- Cough
- Bleeding

- Nausea/vomiting
- Seizures
- Mental status changes

Diagnostic Tests

Hodgkin lymphoma
- Biopsy of the affected lymph node
- CT scan: chest and abdomen
- Positron emission tomographic (PET) imaging

Non-Hodgkin lymphoma
- Biopsy of the affected lymph node
- Bone marrow biopsy
- Laboratory tests
- CT scan: chest and abdomen
- Magnetic resonance imaging (MRI)
- Gallium studies
- Bone scans
- PET imaging
- Microarray analysis

Treatment

Hodgkin and non-Hodgkin lymphoma
- Chemotherapy
- Radiation (localized)

Nursing Interventions and Complications

The nurse should consistently assess for fatigue and malaise with the HL and NHL patient. Encourage the patient to verbalize what he or she feels and assist with ADLs. A diet high in carbohydrates and fluids are necessary as weight loss is persistent with these disease processes. Encourage the patient to take frequent naps and rest when appropriate. If chemotherapy is started, monitor nausea and vomiting, offering antiemetics as needed. Oral care is also important because of the possibility of stomatitis. Address psychosocial concerns such as body image disturbance and alopecia as well as feelings of depression/anxiety due to disease and prolonged fatigue. If the patient is receiving radiation, maintain skin integrity keeping skin cool and intact.

> ### CLINICAL ALERT
>
> *Effects of treatment and the risk for infection are central to the management of the patient with HL or NHL. Institute neutropenic precautions when the WBC <500/μL. Given the treatment modalities, skin, oral mucosa, scalp/hair, nails, and diet are important factors that require vigilance by the nurse. Vital sign assessment is crucial and should be checked against the baseline often. If fever presents, the oncologist health care provider should be notified promptly.*

Multiple Myeloma

When there is a proliferation and accumulation of immunoglobulin-secreting cells (plasma cells), plasma cell neoplasm disease or multiple myeloma ensues. Found more in men than women, the average age of presentation is about 71 years. Multiple myeloma (MM) carries a poor prognosis. It is believed that a displacement of chromosome 14 and the deletion of chromosome 13q trigger this hematopoietic malignancy. The malignant cells are found in the bone marrow and osteolytic lesions throughout the body. Osteolytic bone lesions can cause bone pain, hypercalcemia, and pathologic fractures. Bone marrow infiltration causes dark spots known as purpura. In addition, anemia and neutropenia are common. The patient also demonstrates a high susceptibility to infections. In MM, there are two particular proteins that are characteristic to the disease. They are the M protein and the Bence Jones protein. The M protein is found when electrophoresis is done and the Bence Jones is found in the urine, presenting as proteinuria.

Clinical Manifestations

- Neurologic manifestations presenting as neuropathy
- Spinal cord compression
- Anemia

- Weight loss
- Fatigue
- Pallor
- Deep aching bone pain
- Hepatosplenomegaly
- Confusion
- Recurrent infections
- Renal failure
- Azotemia

Diagnostic Tests

The classic presentation of multiple myeloma is plasmacytosis, lytic bone lesions, and either the presence of the M protein or the Bence Jones protein.

- Presenting symptoms
- Laboratory tests: calcium, electrolytes, erythrocyte sedimentation rate (ESR)
- Bone marrow aspiration
- Bone scans
- X-rays

Treatment

- Chemotherapy
- Thalidomide with corticoidsteroids
- Bortezomib
- Stem cell transplant
- Localized radiation

Nursing Interventions and Complications

The nurse must monitor the patient for cardiac sequelae to hypercalcemia. Because of the accumulation of proteins, renal failure should be a priority assessment. Signs of azotemia or uremia, edema, changes in LOC, and vital signs are important. Nurses should also promptly assess and intervene when the patient is in pain. Assist with comfort modalities, use of narcotics/analgesics, guided imagery and other relaxation techniques. Assess the patient for skin integrity and oral mucosa integrity and institute safeguards to prevent falls given the weakened skeletal system. A diet high in protein and vitamins is warranted. Encourage foods from home. Monitor WBC counts and institute neutropenic precautions when the WBC $<500/\mu L$.

CLINICAL ALERT

Infection management is paramount. Report fevers promptly to the health care provider. Safeguard patient from visitors who are sick and institute safety precautions: seizures, neutropenia, aspiration, and falling as necessary.

REVIEW QUESTIONS

1. A patient with anemia comes to the outpatient clinic complaining of shortness of breath and chest pain. According to the priority of care, what would the nurse do first?

    A. Assess vital signs

    B. Draw bloods

    C. Listen to lung sounds

    D. Assess patient's skin

2. What would be the priority intervention for a patient that has recently been admitted with sickle cell crisis?

    A. Access IV line

    B. Administer pain medication

    C. Review medication orders: pain

    D. Provide reassurance to patient

3. The nurse understands concepts of neutropenia in a patient with leukemia and a WBC <4000 to be:

    A. Placing the patient under reverse isolation

    B. Cohorting the patient with another patient with similar diagnosis

    C. Calling the provider and asking for an extension to the IV lock

    D. Allowing visitors because the patient wants plenty of company

4. The nurse is picking up an order that requires administration of an iron supplement for a patient with anemia. The iron supplement as per the pharmacy is given via injection. Which of the following injections is the correct technique for a drug in this classification?

    A. Intramuscular (IM)

    B. Subcutaneous (SC)

    C. Z-track

    D. Intradermal

5. Which of the following *priority* precautions should the nurse include in the nursing care plan for a neutropenic client with leukemia?

    A. Have the client use a soft toothbrush and electric shaver, avoid using enemas, and watch for signs of bleeding

    B. Put on a mask, gown, and gloves when entering the client's room

    C. Provide a clear liquid, low-sodium diet

    D. Eliminate fresh fruits and veggies, avoid enemas and practice frequent hand washing

Suggested Readings

Christoulas D, Terpos E, Dimopoulos M. Pathogenesis and management of myeloma bone disease. *Expert Rev Hematol.* 2009;2(4):385-398.

Hoppe RT, Advani RH, Ai WZ, et al. NCCN Hodgkin Lymphoma. Hodgkin lymphoma. *J Natl Compr Canc Netw.* 2011;9:1020-1058.

Ignatavicius D, Workman ML. *Medical-Surgical Nursing: Patient Centered Collaborative Care.* 7th ed. St. Louis, MO: Elsevier; 2013.

LeMone P, Burke K, Bostick J. *Clinical Handbook for Medical-surgical Nursing: Critical Thinking in Patient Care.* 5th ed. Upper Saddle River, NJ: Pearson; 2012.

Macdougall IC. New anemia therapies: translating novel strategies from bench to bedside. *Am J Kidney Dis.* 2012;59(3):444-451.

Mason J, Griffiths M. Molecular diagnosis of leukemia. *Expert Rev Mol Diagn.* 2012; 12(5):511-526.

Niscola P, Tendas A, Scaramucci L, et al. Pain in malignant hematology. *Expert Rev Hematol.* 2011;4(1):81-93.

Porth CM. *Essentials of Pathophysiology.* 3rd ed. Philadelphia, PA: Wolters Kluwer Health, Lippincott Williams & Wilkins; 2011.

Rebora P, Czene K, Antolini L, et al. Are chronic myeloid leukemia patients more at risk for second malignancies? A population-based study. *Am J Epidemiol.* 2010; 172(9):1028-1033.

Scudder L. Sickle cell disease management in the emergency department: what every emergency nurse should know. *J Emerg Nurs.* 2011;37:241-345.

Silverberg DS, Wexler D, Iaina A, Schwartz D. Anemia, chronic renal disease and chronic heart failure: the cardiorenal anemia syndrome. *Transfusion Alter Transfusion Med.* 2009;10(4):189-196.

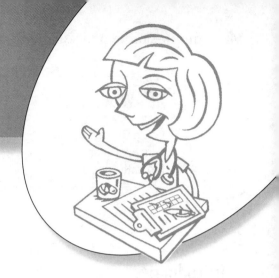

chapter **11**

Cancer

LEARNING OBJECTIVES

At the end of this chapter, the reader/student will be able to:

● Describe the physiologic changes that occur in cancer at the cellular level

● Explain the various types of cancer, including lung, colorectal, pancreatic, liver, prostate, breast, ovarian, uterine, and skin

● Differentiate between the clinical manifestations of the types of cancer

● Describe the nursing care and complications of the types of cancer

Introduction

Cancer is the uncontrolled growth of abnormal cells in the body. Cancerous cells, also called malignant cells, may be the result of cellular, genetic immunologic, and environmental factors. Carcinogenesis is the transformation of normal cells into cancer cells and it is a complex process. At the start of the process, a single genetic change occurs in a normal cell and alters the cell growth and function and the altered cell continues to undergo malignant changes. Normally, there are genes that regulate cell growth, and tumor suppression genes inhibit cellular growth and are called proto-oncogenes. When these proto-oncogenes mutate, they become oncogenes and uncontrolled cell growth occurs.

There are internal (endogenous) and external (exogenous) factors that may result in a malignant process. The endogenous factors are age; specific gene abnormalities, which may be spontaneous or inherited; and immunologic deficiencies. The exogenous factors are tobacco, radiation, certain chemicals that are known to cause cellular damage such as benzene, creosote, and many others, and certain infections such as the human papilloma virus, hepatitis B and C, Epstein-Barr virus, and HIV. Cancer may affect any part of the body, and prognosis depends on the site, how early the cancer is discovered, and if the cancer has metastasized (or spread) to other sites. Metastasis is the major cause of death related to cancer. Cancer cells are different from normal cells in that they lack adhesiveness or the ability to stay with other cells and they break away easily from the tumor and invade surrounding tissue. There are many types of cancer and they are classified according to the cell where the cancer originated from. Carcinoma is a malignant tumor of epithelial cells, and sarcoma is a malignant tumor of connective cells.

Colon Cancer

Cancer of the large bowel (colon and rectum), also called colorectal cancer, is the most common neoplasm of the gastrointestinal tract and the second most common cancer mortality in the United States. Early detection may lead to a much improved outcome. Adenocarcinoma (malignant tumor arising from a glandular organ) accounts for more than 95% of malignancies of the colon and rectum. There is stepwise progression from normal tissue to cancer in the colon and it is best described that when adenomatous polyps are found in the colon, they are at great risk of changing to cancer unless removed. These polyps increase with advancing age and develop in at least 40% of the population. Dietary and environmental factors have been implicated as causes in the development of colon cancer. Diets high in fat and red meat have been linked to colon cancer whereas diets high in fiber, fruits, and vegetable appears to protect against colon cancer. Routine colonoscopies after age 50 years may result in finding these polyps and removing them before the malignant change occurs. There is a type of cancer that is inherited, and genetic testing will determine if a family member has the gene. There are also several genetic mutations among the Ashkenazi Jews that place them at a higher risk of developing colon cancer. Those who have a history of inflammatory bowel disease such as Crohn disease and ulcerative colitis are also at a higher risk for colon cancer. Treatment for colorectal cancer is surgical resection of the cancer, which may result in the person having a colostomy if much of the colon is removed. Chemotherapy may be given even if it is thought that the cancerous tumor has been removed, as a prophylactic measurement. If the colon cancer has metastasized, chemotherapy may be given as a palliative measure as the overall survival rate is 6 months and with best supportive care to 2 years. Improvement in screening for colorectal cancer will prevent many cancers and allow for early treatment, with a greatly improved prognosis (Table 11–1).

Clinical Manifestations

Many patients are asymptomatic. Some presenting symptoms are abdominal cramping or pain, change in bowel habits (constipation, diarrhea, or narrowing of stool), rectal bleeding, dark stools or obvious blood in stool, weakness and fatigue, weight loss, and anemia. If metastasis has occurred, there may be enlarged lymph nodes, pain in liver, and respiratory problems if in lung.

TABLE 11–1 Prophylactic Surgeries in Surgical Oncology	
Prophylactic Surgery	**Potential Indications**
Bilateral mastectomy	*BRCA1* or *BRCA2* mutation
	Atypical hyperplasia or lobular carcinoma in situ
	Familial breast cancer
Bilateral oophorectomy	*BRCA1* mutation
	Familial ovarian cancer
	Hereditary nonpolyposis colorectal cancer
	Hysterectomy for endometrial cancer
	Colon resection for colon cancer
Thyroidectomy	*RET* protooncogene mutation
	Multiple endocrine neoplasia type 2A (MEN 2A)
	Multiple endocrine neoplasia type 2B (MEN 2B)
	Familial non-MEN medullay thyroid carcinoma (FMTC)
Total proctocolectomy	Familial adenomatous polyposis (FAP) or antigen-presenting cell (APC) mutation
	Ulcerative colitis
	Hereditary nonpolyposis colorectal cancer (HNPCC) germ-line mutation

Reproduced with permission from Doherty G. *Current Diagnosis and Treatment Surgery*. 13th ed. New York: McGraw-Hill; 2009, table 44-1.

Diagnostic Tests

Complete blood count (CBC), liver function tests, fecal occult blood test, colonoscopy with biopsy, computed tomographic (CT) scan to evaluate for metastasis, chest x-ray, magnetic resonance imaging (MRI), and endoscopic ultrasonography may be used to evaluate extent of rectal cancers.

Treatment

Resection of the primary tumor in the colon or rectum is the treatment of choice, with regional dissection of at least 12 lymph nodes to determine the staging of the cancer. The stages range from I to IV, with stage I having best prognosis and stage IV metastatic disease, which 20% of patients have at diagnosis. Chemotherapy and radiation therapy are the course of treatment.

Nursing Intervention and Complications

Prepare patient for abdominal surgery with bowel cleansing (laxatives, enemas) to suppress bacterial growth. Teach the patients about the planned surgery and what to expect such as nasogastric tube, a possible colostomy. Support the patient when fearful and anxious. Postsurgical care includes continued assessment of close fluid and electrolyte balance, maintain adequate ventilation, assess patient for a paralytic ileus, and support early ambulation. If metastasis is discovered during surgery and prognosis is poor, support the patient and the family and encourage verbalization of fears. Administer chemotherapy as ordered. If the patient has a colostomy, teach family about the care needed and encourage the patient to assume care as soon as possible. Complications may occur because of the extensive nature of the surgery, such as infection, bleeding, anastomosis leakage, and possible fistula development. If extensive lymph nodes were removed, nerve pathways may have been affected, causing urinary lack of control. Long-term complications are related to disease recurrence and metastatic disease.

CLINICAL ALERT

The majority of patients with metastatic disease do not have curable disease. In the absence of other treatment, the median survival is 6 months. The goals of therapy are to slow tumor progression to extend life for as long as possible.

Pancreatic Cancer

Pancreatic cancer is a malignant disease involving the head of the pancreas, the distal common bile duct, and the duodenum together because they are virtually indistinguishable clinically. The pancreas lies behind the stomach and in front of the first and second lumbar vertebrae. The head of the pancreas lies within the curve of the duodenum and the tail lies near the spleen. More than 85% of cases are ductal adenocarcinomas. Approximately 75% of these cancers develop in the head of the pancreas and the 25% are found in the body or the tail. Pancreatic cancer ranks as the fourth leading cause of cancer death in the United States. This pancreatic exocrine cancer is rarely curable and has an overall 5-year survival rate of less than 5.5%. Only 7% of pancreatic cancers are localized when diagnosed; 26% have already spread to the lymph nodes and

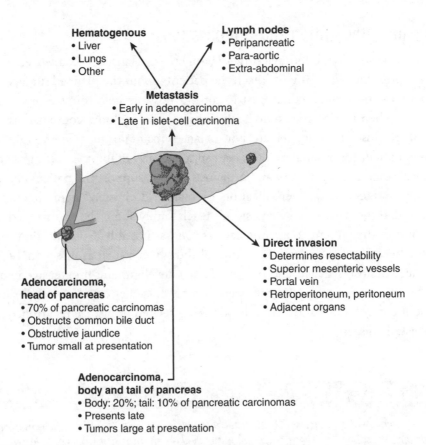

Hematogenous
• Liver
• Lungs
• Other

Lymph nodes
• Peripancreatic
• Para-aortic
• Extra-abdominal

Metastasis
• Early in adenocarcinoma
• Late in islet-cell carcinoma

Direct invasion
• Determines resectability
• Superior mesenteric vessels
• Portal vein
• Retroperitoneum, peritoneum
• Adjacent organs

Adenocarcinoma, head of pancreas
• 70% of pancreatic carcinomas
• Obstructs common bile duct
• Obstructive jaundice
• Tumor small at presentation

Adenocarcinoma, body and tail of pancreas
• Body: 20%; tail: 10% of pancreatic carcinomas
• Presents late
• Tumors large at presentation

FIGURE 11–1 • Pancreatic cancer: location and pattern of spread. (Reproduced with permission from Chandrasoma P, et al. *Concise Pathology*. 3rd ed. New York: McGraw-Hill; 1997, figure 15-9.)

53% have already metastasized. Pancreatic cancer is rare before middle age and increases with age. It occurs more frequently in men. The cause is not known, but cigarette smoking is believed to be a causative factor, in addition to a possible hereditary component. A diet high in fruits and vegetables shows evidence of protection against the disease. Often the disease is advanced because of vague symptoms at first as well as there is no capsule surrounding the pancreas to contain growth and spreading of the disease. After diagnosis, the usual survival time is only 18–20 months. Male-to-female ratio is 13:1 (Figure 11–1).

Clinical Manifestations

Upper abdominal pain that may radiate to the back (pain worse as cancer progresses), anorexia, weight loss, weakness, fatigue, dark urine, clay-colored stools, jaundice, hyperglycemia, and unexplained increase in clotting tendencies.

Diagnostic Tests

CA 19-9; abdominal ultrasonography; CT or MRI scan; endoscopic retrograde cholangiopancreatography (ERCP); positron emission tomographic (PET) scan; fine-needle biopsy; CBC; serum glucose; serum amylase; and occult blood are generally used to confirm tests.

Treatment

Treatment is abdominal exploration, and the most radical surgery is the removal of the pancreas, duodenum, distal bile duct, proximal jejunum, partial gastrectomy, and removal of regional lymph nodes and is called a Whipple procedure. This procedure is only attempted if there is a possibility of a cure as it is a very complex surgery and requires a very long recovery period. In most cases, the options are palliative care such as placement of stents in the bile duct, radiation therapy, and chemotherapy with gemcitabine as there has been improved response rate with this drug. Other chemotherapy has been disappointing with metastatic disease, but may be used palliatively in pancreatic cancer that cannot be resected and is only confined to the pancreas.

Nursing Interventions and Complications

Pain management and treatment for it; fluid and electrolyte balance; assess nutrition and elimination by monitoring laboratory values for serum albumin and protein levels, weigh patient daily; if surgery is performed, closely monitor patient because of the complexity of the operation; assess for jaundice and obstruction due to large tumors; administer chemotherapy as ordered; provide patient and family education regarding management of pain, the ongoing challenges and side effects of treatments; provide emotional support for patient and family, and provide palliative and end-of-life care. The complications are surgical infection, obstruction, excruciating pain, and ultimately death.

CLINICAL ALERT

The patient with pancreatic cancer may also develop diabetes mellitus because of damage to the pancreas. Surgical complications may include abscess and gastric and biliary leakage from the site of anastomosis. Carcinoma of the pancreas has a poor prognosis and only about 2%–5% of patients live to 5 years after diagnosis. Nurses must provide excellent postsurgical care and prepare and support the patient and family through palliative and end-of-life care.

Prostate Cancer

Cancer of the prostate is the most common cancer in adult men in the United States and the second leading cause of cancer-related deaths. There are approximately 218,000 new cases of prostate cancer each year in the United States. As was described in the chapter on reproduction, the prostate is a gland consisting of three lobes that surround the neck of the male bladder and neck of the urethra. Cancer of the prostate is a malignant tumor that is almost always an adenocarcinoma. It occurs most often in older men.

Although 40% of men older than age 50 years are found to have prostatic carcinoma, most are small and contained within the prostate gland. The mean age of diagnosis is 71 years and most are diagnosed over age 65 years. Factors that may affect the development of prostate cancer are hormonal changes in testosterone levels. It has also been thought that certain viruses, such as a strain of cytomegalovirus, can produce malignant changes. Prostate cancer can spread locally or metastasize through the lymphatic system to the lungs, liver, brain, and bone.

Screening for prostate-specific antigen (PSA) in men older than age 50 years can find cancers early when it is localized and can be easily treated with PSA levels <10 ng/mL. In untreated patients with prostate cancer, the level of PSA correlates with the volume and staging of the disease, and approximately 98% of metastatic disease will have elevated PSA in excess of 40 ng/mL (Figure 11–2).

Clinical Manifestations

As the tumor grows, the prostate enlarges, causing urinary problems, such as difficulty urinating or urinary obstruction; decreased urinary stream; erectile dysfunction; bloody semen or hematuria; and focal nodules or areas of induration within the prostate (palpated by health care provider). In advanced disease, patients may have bone pain and lymph node enlargement.

Diagnostic Tests

PSA levels; blood urea nitrogen (BUN), creatinine levels, urinalysis, alkaline phosphatase (elevated in bony metastasis); transrectal ultrasonography–guided biopsy; MRI; and radionuclide bone scan can be used to confirm diagnosis.

Treatment

Treatment for prostate cancer ranges from hormone therapy to block testosterone production, such as leuprolide acetate (Lupron), goserelin acetate

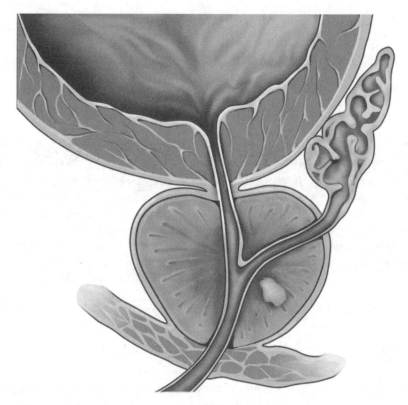

FIGURE 11–2 • T stages of prostate cancer. T1—Clinically inapparent tumor, neither palpable nor visible by imaging. (Data from AJCC, http://seer.cancer.gov/statfacts/html/prost.html. Figure © Memorial Sloan-Kettering Cancer Center Medical Graphics, used with permission.)

(Zoladex) or estrogen therapy, to radiation treating local tumors with either external radiation or insertion of radioactive seeds, to several surgical options of prostatectomy or removal of the prostate. When testosterone suppression is necessary and the hormonal methods do not work, bilateral orchiectomy may be necessary.

Nursing Interventions and Complications

Preoperative care preparing the patient, which includes a bowel preparation; educating the patient and family on what to expect postsurgically; providing postoperative care to the perineal wound; assess urinary drainage and bleeding; treat bladder spasms; prepare for possible fecal incontinence because the surgery can cause relaxation of the perineal musculature; prepare for sexual problems such as erectile dysfunction; and provide emotional support and spend time with the patient who is dealing with the fear of cancer diagnosis and loss of sexuality. Complications of a radical prostatectomy may be hemorrhage, urinary and bowel incontinence, leakage from the surgical site, and metastasis to other organs such as lymph nodes, bowel, bones, liver, and lungs.

> ## CLINICAL ALERT
>
> *Cancer can extend beyond the capsule boundaries and spread to the lymphatic and vascular system. The common places of metastasis are the bones, pelvis, spine, femur, and ribs and may involve the lung, liver, and kidney in late disease. Nurses must be alert to patient with prostate with other complaints as it may be indicative of metastasis. One in 6 men will be diagnosed with prostate cancer, but only 1 in 30 will die of the disease.*

Breast Cancer

Breast cancer is the most common cancer among women. The incidence of breast carcinoma continues to increase partly due to the aging population and partly due to better diagnostic testing. Only about 10% of breast cancers are inherited, which means that two or more first-degree relatives have had breast cancer before the age of 50 years. Other risk factors are family history of bilateral disease, a combination of breast cancer and another epithelial cancer such as ovarian cancer, family member with male breast cancer, and an Ashkenazi Jewish heritage. Mutations in the *BRCA1* and *BRCA2* genes are present in high-risk families. The development of noninherited breast cancer occurs first when there is a change in cell structure and then there is another change in the cell that causes it to become malignant. Excessive amounts of estrogen play a part such as when a women gets her period before the age of 12 years and goes through menopause after age 55 years. Risk is also greater in women who have never been pregnant or have their first child after age 30 years.

Postmenopausal hormone replacement therapy and use of oral contraceptives have shown that long-term use may show a higher increase of breast cancer. Obesity has been linked to breast cancer as androgens in fat cells can be converted to estrogens, thereby increasing estrogens in the body. Women have a one in eight chance of developing breast cancer in their lifetime. Breast cancer accounts for about a third of all cancer found in women and about 15% of all cancer-related deaths. Incidence and mortality rates are highest in the United States and Western Europe. In the United States, Caucasian women have the highest rate of breast cancer.

Prognosis of the disease depends on whether the disease is localized or invasive, grade of the disease, lymph node involvement, tumor size, and if the tumor is estrogen/progesterone sensitive and genetic markers. Tumors arise from the epithelial cells of either the ductal or lobular tissue of the breast. Early-stage cancer has no symptoms and may be detected on physical examination or by a mammogram or breast sonogram when approximately 35%–50% of cancers are discovered. With more advanced disease, a tumor can be palpated that is fixed to the chest wall versus benign tumors, which are well defined and movable. The skin surrounding the malignant tumor may be dimpled and the nipple may be retracted. The skin may look like an orange peel with large pores, which indicates that there is lymphatic obstruction from the tumor growth with resulting edema. Sixty percent of breast cancers are in the upper outer quadrant of the breast. Breast carcinoma is staged like other cancers from stages I to IV. Breast cancer can spread to the bone, lung, liver, and brain. A type of breast carcinoma called inflammatory carcinoma is the most malignant form of breast cancer and consists of a rapidly growing painful mass, and no distinct mass can be palpated as it infiltrates the breast diffusely and is often treated as an infection. It is invasive and infiltrates the lymphatic system. Metastasis occurs early and widely, and is rarely curable. This type of breast cancer only affects 3% of women. Currently, the use of vitamin D is thought to lower the risk of developing breast cancer (Figure 11–3).

Clinical Manifestations

Seventy percent of patients present with a breast lump. Less frequent signs are breast pain, nipple discharge, erosion, retraction, enlargement, itching of the nipple and redness, generalized hardness of breast. Back or bone pain, jaundice, or weight loss may be the result of disease that has already metastasized.

Diagnostic Tests

Sedimentation rate, serum alkaline phosphatase, CEA 125, and CA15-3 or CA27-29 (for metastasis and recurrent breast cancer), chest x-ray, CT scan of liver; PET scan, biopsy of breast, ultrasonography of breast, mammography, MRI, and cytology of nipple discharge or cyst fluid can confirm diagnoses.

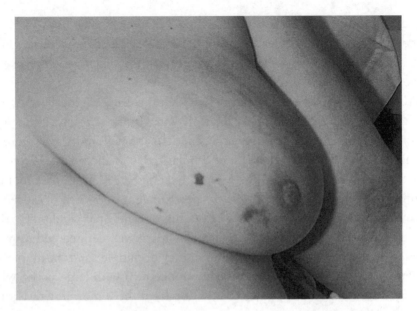

FIGURE 11–3 • Photographs of inflammatory breast cancer. Subtle erythematous blush and edema in inflammatory breast cancer. (Reproduced with permission from Hoffman B, et al. *William's Gynecology.* 2nd ed. New York: McGraw-Hill; 2012, figure 12-16. Photographs contributed by Dr. Marilyn Leitch.)

Treatment

Treatment may be curative or palliative depending on the type of cancer and stage at diagnosis. Surgery may include resection of the lump conserving the breast, to a mastectomy, and removal of lymph nodes to determine metastasis. Additional treatments are radiation therapy, chemotherapy, endocrine therapy for hormone-receptive breast cancers with estrogen-receptor antagonists/ agonist such as tamoxifen, which decrease the risk of breast cancer in the other breast but can cause endometrial cancer and thromboembolic events. Frequent pelvic sonograms can be taken to determine if the endometrium (lining in the uterus) is thickened, and the nurse should be alert to any thrombus forming. Palliative treatment such as radiotherapy and bisphosphonates such as zole- dronic acid are given for advanced metastatic breast cancer patients.

Nursing Interventions and Complications

Nursing care aims at helping patients with breast cancer with the various treat- ment options and surgical interventions. The diagnosis of cancer is very trau- matic, and nurses encourage the patients to discuss the grieving process, body image alteration, and change in sexuality.

Nurses educate and prepare the patient for surgery and for the reconstructive surgery (called a TRAM flap, which is an extensive surgery that often is done along with the surgery today), and what in the plan the patient can expect. Managing postoperative pain, preventing infections, and promoting mobility is important. Nurses instruct the patient and family on wound care, exercise, and signs of infection; arrange follow-up appointment with oncologist or for radiation therapy; and initiate referral to organizations such as Reach for Recovery (where other women who have had breast cancer provide support to those newly diagnosed). Explain what to expect from chemotherapy such as "chemo brain" and assure that among the symptoms, many will resolve once chemotherapy has ended. Encourage good nutrition.

CLINICAL ALERT

Patients must be monitored long term in order to detect recurrences and to observe the opposite breast for a secondary carcinoma. Local and distant recurrences occur most frequently in the first 2–5 years. Men must also monitor for breast cancer as the prognosis is poor for men than women. Survival rate for men is 58% and for women 38% in the 5-year mark. Patients who have advanced cancer must receive meticulous palliative care from nurses and support in preparations for death.

Ovarian Cancer

Ovarian cancer is the ninth most common cancer in women and the fifth leading cause of cancer death in women. Prevalence and mortality rates are highest in Caucasian women. Malignant neoplasms of the ovaries occur at all ages, including infancy and childhood. In the United States, ovarian cancer has the highest mortality rate of gynecologic cancers. There are about 24,000 new cases of ovarian cancer diagnosed each year and more than 13,000 deaths in the United States. Ninety percent of ovarian cancer is sporadic and not inherited, although family history, increasing age, nulliparity (never having delivered a child), early menarche, late menopause, use of hormone replacement therapy, and a history of breast cancer are known to add to the risk of developing ovarian cancer. The genes *BRCA1* and *BRCA2* are inherited and indicate a high likelihood of developing ovarian and breast cancer.

Eating a diet high in fat, using talc, and using fertility drugs may also put a woman at risk for developing ovarian cancer. Women older than age 50 years are at malignant epithelial cell tumors and those younger than age 20 years with ovarian cancer usually have malignant germ cell tumors. There are several theories as to why ovarian cancer occurs: (1) possible repeated ovulation disrupts the ovaries, which leads to a malignant change; (2) persistent stimulation of the ovary by the pituitary stimulation of luteinizing hormone (LH) and follicle-stimulating hormone (FSH) may be carcinogenic; and (3) processing of chemical carcinogens in the local ovarian environment could lead to cancer. Currently, there are no available effective screening tests to detect ovarian cancer early. Recently, the CA 125 and HE 4 (ROMA) have been used together if an ovarian mass is found on ultrasonography or through a pelvic examination to determine if the ovarian mass is benign or malignant. In a postmenopausal woman, when ovaries are palpated during an examination, it becomes highly suspicious for a pathology.

Ovaries normally are very small in postmenopausal women and are not palpated. Ovarian cancer is difficult to detect in its early stages as many of the initial symptoms are vague, and even with advanced treatment modalities, the 5-year survival rate is only about 46%.

Almost 70% of patients have already reached advanced-stage disease at the time they seek help. Treatment is surgical debulking of the tumor, an omentectomy, total abdominal hysterectomy, and bilateral salpingo-oophorectomy (removal of the fallopian tubes and both ovaries); combination chemotherapy and radiation is also used.

Clinical Manifestations

Unfortunately, in malignant disease of the ovary, there are only mild nonspecific symptoms, such as pelvic pressure. Enlargement of the ovary is usually detected during a routine gynecologic examination. Women who have more advanced disease may have abdominal pain, bloating, a palpable mass, and ascites.

Diagnostic Tests

Once a mass is detected, a lab CA 125 test >35 units indicates that the tumor is probably malignant; transvaginal ultrasonography; presence of symptoms; and surgery with biopsy.

Treatment

If an ovarian mass is suspected, surgical evaluation is performed by a gyneco-logic oncologist. Surgery is performed with staging followed by an abdominal hysterectomy, bilateral oophorectomy, and omentectomy along with lymph node removal to determine if the cancer has metastasized. Chemotherapy follows the surgery.

Nursing Interventions and Complications

Nursing care is aimed at teaching the patient regarding their concerns about the diagnostic surgery, and the other therapies such as chemotherapy for ovar-ian cancer. Support and educate the family regarding each step from diagnosis until the final stages if the cancer is higher than grade 1. Include the patient in all decisions.

CLINICAL ALERT

A pelvic mass even a cyst larger than 7.5 cm should be observed for 4–6 weeks to see if it has resolved. If not, surgical intervention with biopsy is indicated. Because of the high mortality of those diagnosed with ovarian cancer, early diagnosis if possible gives the best chance of survival before it has spread. Nurses must know the risks associated with developing ovarian cancer, and those who have relatives with ovarian cancer should be screened frequently and any ovarian mass should be considered suspicious until proven otherwise.

Uterine Cancer

Cancer of the endometrium (uterine cancer) is the most common cancer of the female genital tract. It is most often found in women 50–70 years of age. Endometrial cancer is twice as common as ovarian cancer. Uterine hyperplasia (overgrowth of the endometrial lining) can undergo cancerous changes. Ade-nocarcinoma of the endometrium is higher in obesity, nulliparity, polycystic ovarian syndrome, prolonged anovulation, unopposed estrogen therapy, and extended use of drugs like tamoxifen used in the treatment of breast cancer. Unlike cervical dysplasia (abnormal development of tissue), there is no widely available screening for endometrial hyperplasia. Most women seek medical care for abnormal uterine bleeding. The underlying pathologic process involves overgrowth of the uterine lining in response to an estrogen-dominant hormonal environment. Prompt endometrial sampling of those who report abnormal bleeding will reveal endometrial cancers. Young women with chronic anovulation are at risk for endometrial hyperplasia and can reduce the risk of developing cancer by taking oral contraceptives. The 5-year survival rate with early diagnosis is 80%–85% and with great invasion 66%. Staging of uterine cancer is I–IV. Stage IV involves the bladder, rectum, or outside pelvis.

Clinical Manifestations

Abnormal bleeding is present in 80% of uterine cancers. There may be obstruction of the cervix, with a collection of pus or blood causing lower abdominal pain. Sometimes a Pap test will show atypical endometrial cells, but it is not a good diagnostic tool.

Diagnostic Tests

Endometrial sampling with a suction curette (Pipelle) or a more conclusive test called a hysteroscopy can be used that can localize polyps and other lesions in the endometrial cavity. Vaginal ultrasonography can determine thickness in the endometrium. Pap test, liver tests, and cancer antigen (CA125) may be elevated when intraabdominal disease is present. CT scan and MRI can be used to determine if lymphadenopathy is present.

Treatment

Total hysterectomy and bilateral salpingo-oophorectomy (removal of uterus, ovaries, and fallopian tubes) or lymph node sampling is done and if the cancer is deep in the endometrium, postoperative radiation is indicated. Palliative care in advanced metastatic endometrial cancer may be accomplished with large doses of progestins and weekly megestrol acetate (Megace), which treats anorexia and weight loss from the cancer. The role of chemotherapy alone or with radiation shows only a modest increase in survival.

Nursing Interventions and Complications

Postoperative care after the surgery for cancer is aimed at pain management and prevention of infections and complications. Nurses teach women about the importance of following up immediately when they have abnormal bleeding, especially in the postmenopausal populations, to reduce the fatality rate by identifying endometrial cancer at a stage when it can be treated.

CLINICAL ALERT

Early diagnosis and treatment prevents deaths from advanced disease. It is a slow growing cancer and responsive to treatment if found early.

CASE STUDY

M.J., a woman aged 46, is seen by the nurse practitioner after her husband found a lump in her right breast in the upper outer quadrant. She has never been pregnant. This is the first time in 5 years that she is seeing any health care provider and has never had a mammography.

She is overweight, 199 lbs at height 5′, and states she loves steak, fried food, and foods with a lot of gravy. She does not exercise and her job consists of sitting at a computer all day. She got her first period at age 9 and is still menstruating.

QUESTIONS

1. What are some of M.J.'s risk factors for breast cancer?
2. What other questions would the nurse practitioner ask?
3. Which is the most common site for breast cancer?
4. What tests would the nurse practitioner order for this patient?
5. What behaviors would the nurse practitioner try to modify with this patient?

Suggested Readings

Bergren T, Heuberger R. Vitamin D and breast cancer prevention. *Nurs Womens Health*. 2010;14(5):368-375.

Corall AH, Mulby AG. *Primary Care Medicine*. 4th ed. Philadelphia, PA: Lippincott Williams & Wilkins; 2000.

Doenges ME, Moorhouse MF, Murr AC. *Nursing Diagnosis Manual*. Philadelphia, PA: F.A. Davis; 2010.

Domino F. *The 5 Minute Clinical Consults 2011*. 19th ed. Philadelphia, PA: Wolters Kluwer/Lippincott Williams & Wilkins; 2010.

Goroll AH, Mulley AG. *Primary Care Medicine*. 4th ed. Philadelphia, PA: Lippincott Williams & Wilkins; 2000.

Greco KE, Nail LM, Kendall J, Cartwright J, Massecar DC. Mammography decision making in older women with breast cancer family history. *J Nurs Scholarsh*. 2010; 42(3):348-355.

Guyton AC, Hall JE. *Textbook of Medical Physiology*. 9th ed. Philadelphia, PA: W.B. Saunders; 1996.

Kelley WN. *Textbook of Internal Medicine*. 3rd ed. Philadelphia, PA: Lippincott-Raven; 1992.

Marx J, Hockberger R, Walls R. *Rosen's Emergency Medicine*. 7th ed. St. Louis, MO: Mosby; 2009.

McPhee SJ, Papadakis MA, Rabow MW. *2011 Current Medical Diagnosis & Treatment*. New York: McGraw-Hill; 2011.

Phipps WJ, Monhahan FD, Sands JK, Marek JF, Neighbors M. *Medical-Surgical Nursing Health and Illness Perspectives*. 7th ed. St. Louis, MO: Mosby; 2003.

Porth CM. *Essentials of Pathophysiology*. 3rd ed. Philadelphia, PA: Lippincott Williams & Wilkins; 2011.

Professional Guide to Signs and Symptoms. 5th ed. Philadelphia, PA: Lippincott Williams & Wilkins; 2009.

Ratner E, Richter C, Minkin M, Foran-Tuller F. How to talk about sexual issues with cancer patients beginning the dialogue. *Contemp Ob-Gyn*. 2012;57(5):40-51.

Robinson R. Early identification of pancreatic cancer. *Clin Rev*. 2012;22(4):27-33.

Star W, Lommel LL, Shannon MT. *Women's Primary Health Care Protocols for Practice*. 2nd ed. San Francisco, CA: UCSF Nursing Press; 2004.

Taber's Cyclopedic Medical Dictionary. Philadelphia, PA: F.A. Davis; 2009.

Xi T, Kappa G. Women receiving news of a family *BRCA1/2* mutation: messages of fear and empowerment. *J Nurs Scholarsh*. 2010;42(4):367-378.

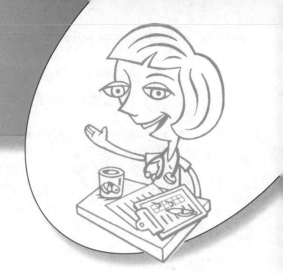

Autoimmune System

LEARNING OBJECTIVES

At the end of this chapter, the reader/student will be able to:

- Describe the physiology of the normal immune system
- Outline the possible etiologies for autoimmune disease
- Discuss nursing care of patients with select autoimmune diseases
- Compare the pathophysiology of HIV infection and AIDS
- Explain the pathologic changes that occur with systemic lupus erythematosus (SLE)

KEY WORDS

Human Immunodeficiency Virus
Acquired Immune Deficiency
Syndrome (AIDS)

Systemic Lupus
Erythematosus

Introduction

In the normal healthy individual, the immune response is a protective one, but the protection depends on an intact immune system. The human body has the ability to resist almost all types of organisms or toxins that tend to damage the tissues and organs. This capacity is called immunity. Much of immunity is *acquired* that develops after the body is first attacked by a bacterial disease or toxin. Additional immunity is called *innate immunity* and results from phagocytosis of bacteria, resistance of the skin to invasion by organisms, and the presence of certain chemical compounds in the blood that attack foreign organisms and toxins and destroy them. Some names of the chemical compounds are lysozymes, the complement complex that is a system of about 20 proteins that can be activated to destroy bacteria, and natural killer lymphocytes that can recognize and destroy foreign cells, tumor cells, and even some infected cells. *Acquired immunity* results either from exposure of an antigen such as viruses and toxins and when the intact immune system has the ability of developing antibodies to these potentially lethal bacteria or toxins or through immunizations that expose the person to small amounts of the toxin so that the body builds antibodies that are globulins to the disease or virus, thereby protecting the body from getting the disease. This is also called B-cell immunity, because the B lymphocytes produce the antibodies. The second type of acquired immunity is achieved through large numbers of activated lymphocytes that specifically destroy the foreign agent. This type is called *cell-mediated immunity* or *T-cell immunity*, because the activated lymphocytes are T lymphocytes. The lymphocytes that are destined to become these T lymphocytes first migrate to and are preprocessed in the thymus gland, which is why they are called T lymphocytes. Proteins on the surface of lymphocytes that enhance immune recognition are called CD4 molecules.

Immune cells that express the CD4 molecule are also known as helpers to T cells. The immune system is very complex. In healthy individuals who have also been immunized against potentially lethal diseases, the system functions without the person even being aware of the internal war on organisms that is occurring in their body. In immunocompromised patients and the elderly, these normal defenses do not protect them as well as in the healthy individual, which results in susceptibility to a variety of diseases. There are many diseases produced called autoimmune diseases and occur when the body's normal tolerance of the antigens on its own cell (autoantigens or self-antigens) is disrupted. Some conditions that can suppress the immune system are nephrotic syndrome, burns, severe liver disease, cancer, alcoholism, diabetes, infections, and lymphomas. Autoimmunity or again the formations of antibodies against self-tissue can be influenced by genetic, hormonal, viral, and environmental factors.

Some of these diseases, for example, are ulcerative colitis, autoimmune thyroiditis (Graves), myasthenia gravis, and multiple sclerosis.

Human Immunodeficiency Virus

HIV is caused by a retrovirus. The retroviruses HIV-1 and HIV-2 are associated with depletion of the CD4 or helper cell to the T lymphocytes. The virus replicates and uses the CD4 receptors, causing cell death, and results in severe immunodeficiency. HIV is associated with a very unpredictable disease progression, and some patients can have no symptoms for as long as 10 years even though the virus is still detected in their blood. They may experience some slight immunologic alterations. The mode of transmission of HIV is similar to hepatitis B and is spread through certain sexual practices and by parenteral and vertical transmission. Mothers with HIV can transmit the virus to their unborn child. Of those at risk for HIV and who engage in a variety of sexual practices and have sex with multiple partners, only some will actually be infected with HIV. The best available estimates indicate that the risk of HIV transmission with receptive anal intercourse is between 1:100 and 1:30. Worldwide, there are an estimated 33.4 million persons infected with HIV. Once a patient becomes symptomatic with HIV, the number of T4 helper cells can be detected and the virus replicates dramatically. The complications of HIV-related infections and neoplasms affect almost every organ. Immunodeficiency is a direct result of the effects of HIV on the immune cells.

Acquired Immune Deficiency Syndrome (AIDS)

Between exposure with the HIV virus and the development of AIDS, the time can vary as much as 10 years. The development of symptoms may start off as nonspecific, such as generalized lymphadenopathy, fever, fatigue, and night sweats. The symptoms that are specific to HIV infection are hairy leukoplakia of the tongue; disseminated Kaposi sarcoma, which is a rare cancer with lesions appearing on the skin, mucous membranes, mouth, tongue, sclera, and may also affect the internal organs; and another common complication, *Pneumocystis pneumonia* infection. These are all opportunistic infections related to immunodeficiency and the low CD4 count. The organisms that cause these infections are harmless to people with intact immune systems, but these highly compromised patients can die of such complications because every aspect of their immune system is dysfunctional.

The virus easily enters and replicates and overwhelms the patient. The person with HIV/AIDS may experience one or more infections at the same time, producing many challenges. The infections may be fungal, and others might be caused by protozoa, bacteria, and certain cancers. The central nervous system can be affected and the diagnosis of AIDS dementia as well as neurologic deficits such as aphasia and hemiparesis can occur in advance AIDS. Often in the literature, HIV and AIDS are used interchangeably, but HIV is the virus and AIDS is when the virus takes over the immune system and causes all of the symptoms that can affect every system in the body and lead to death if not treated with antiviral medications. There are 1.2 million people living with HIV in the United States. (Figures 12–1 and 12–2).

Clinical Manifestations

Fever, lymphadenopathy, diarrhea, perirectal pain, dysphagia, cutaneous lesions, possible dementia, malignancies such as (Kaposi sarcoma, lymphoma), dysphagia, weight loss, blindness, pneumonia, and multiple fungal and bacterial opportunistic infections affecting the lungs, heart, endocrine system, liver, skin, oral cavity, and in women cervical dysplasia and pelvic inflammatory disease.

Diagnostic Tests

Enzyme-linked immunosorbent assay (ELISA) HIV test including antibodies and antigen detection; CD4 lymphocyte count; complete blood count (CBC) with differential; serum chemistry; hepatitis A, B, and C and syphilis test

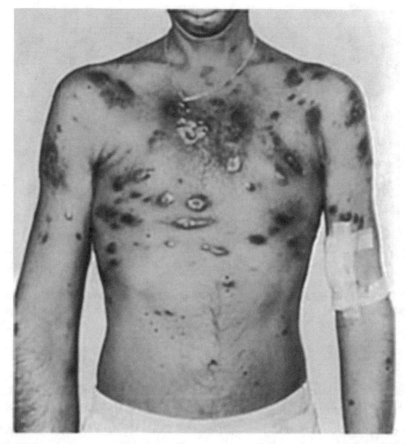

FIGURE 12–1 • Kaposi sarcoma, disseminated, in a patient with AIDS. Note the presence of multiple elevated white skin lesions. (Reproduced with permission from Chandrasoma P, et al. *Concise Pathology*. 3rd ed. New York: McGraw-Hill; 1997, figure 7-5.)

(immunocompromised HIV patients easily get other infections and the sexual-risk behavior causes other disease); urine or cervical screening for sexually transmitted infections; and chest x-ray are generally performed.

Treatment

Prevention should be stressed to all at-risk patients. There are many antiviral medications that are used in combination, and they decrease the viral load of HIV with the intent of preventing overwhelming AIDS. Usually, the treatment regime is based on the CD4 count.

The antivirals can be used for prophylaxis for opportunistic infections and malignancies. If the patient has complications of HIV, the system that

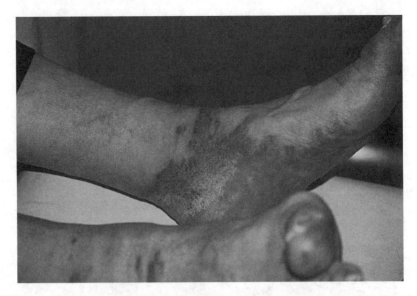

FIGURE 12–2 • KS on the foot in a man with AIDS in the 1990s. Note the lesion. (Reproduced with permission from Wolff K, Johnson R. *Fitzpatrick's Color Atlas and Synopsis of Clinical Dermatology.* 6th ed. New York: McGraw-Hill; 2009, figure 20-18.)

is affected should be treated (e.g., pneumocystic pneumonia is treated with antibiotics), but the antiviral medications should also be used to try to prevent other complications by decreasing the viral load. Treatment regimes are constantly changing and there are new and experimental treatments. Some of the antivirals are protease inhibitors, and some are nonnucleoside reverse transcriptase inhibitors. They prevent replication of the virus with different pharmacologic methods. The introduction of highly active antiretroviral therapy has transformed a rapidly progressive life-threatening illness to a chronic manageable condition. There are antivirals, although prolonging life have many side effects associated with their use. The description of the pharmacodynamics of the antivirals is not for discussion in this book. The hope is that there will be an HIV vaccine developed that would protect against getting the virus.

Nursing Interventions and Complications

Health assessment of patients at risk for HIV should be in a complete nursing history. When a patient has HIV, nurses assess for symptoms and complications of AIDS. Nursing diagnoses are as follows: risk for infection due to the compromised immune system; imbalance of nutrition; fatigue; and ineffective coping of the patient. Nurses also teach patients to prevent being infected with HIV, and if the patient has HIV the nurse teaches the patients about treatment options. The nurse is also expected to carry out the complex treatments of multiple system disease (respiratory management, skin and mucous membrane care), fluid balance, perineal care for diarrhea, and managing fear and anxiety are also part of nursing interventions. The complications are the severe opportunistic infections and the development of cancers such as Kaposi sarcoma, cervical cancer, and non-Hodgkin lymphoma.

CLINICAL ALERT

The more severe opportunistic infections are by Mycobacterium avium *complex that causes persistent high fevers, night sweats, weight loss, abdominal pain, and diarrhea and can be disseminated throughout the body and is a wasting syndrome. Cryptococcosis is a yeast-like fungus found in pigeon droppings, soil, and the environment and can cause central nervous system symptoms of fever, headache, memory changes, vomiting, fatigue, convulsions, and if untreated will cause coma and death from cerebral edema.*

Toxoplasma gondii is found in cats and meats. It causes encephalitis and if disseminated, infections can lead to headache, confusion, delirium, fever, vomiting, hemiparesis, seizures, and loss of vision. Viral infection by cytomegalovirus (CMV), one of which is the herpes virus, can cause disseminated disease affecting the brain, liver, and lungs and produce blindness, seizures, deafness, and death. These infections do not infect those with health immune systems but are deadly to those with HIV-AIDS.

Systemic Lupus Erythematosus

Systemic lupus erythematosus (SLE) is a set of clinical disorders involving multiple organ systems. It is characterized by producing autoantibodies, one of which is antinuclear antibodies (ANAs). Because of the autoimmune nature of this disease, it is complicated and there is a wide variation in clinical presentation. The incidence of this inflammatory disease occurs in females 10 times higher than in males. The incidence of SLE is influenced by many factors, including gender, race, and genetic inheritance. The occurrence in white women is 1:1000, but in black women it is increased to 1:250, and usually occurs during the childbearing years. The risk drops off dramatically after menopause. The course of the disease is marked by spontaneous remissions and relapses.

SLE is a chronic inflammatory autoimmune disease (when the body turns against its own antigen on its own cells) and affects primarily the skin, joints, and kidneys; nevertheless, it can affect every organ of the body. Most cases of SLE are idiopathic. It is thought that the B lymphocytes that mature in the bone marrow and play a major role in the body's natural defense may be responsible for causing an increase in the production of antibodies, for which the body has an inappropriate response to the antibodies against itself. Erythema and a butterfly-pattern rash across the cheeks and bridge of nose when the person is exposed to sun may be the first indication of SLE.

Clinical Manifestations

Fever, anorexia, malaise, weight loss, skin lesions, butterfly rash, alopecia, erythema under the nails, joint pain, photosensitivity, fibromyalgia, pleurisy, pneumonia, cardiac arrhythmias or acute or chronic valvular incompetence, mesenteric vasculitis, abdominal pain, psychosis, seizures, strokes, and glomerulonephritis are the most common. Affected organs may range from the skin, eyes, joints, chest, cardiac system, abdomen, neurologic system, and the kidneys.

Diagnostic Tests

Antinuclear antibody test is positive in SLE; a depressed complementary finding is also suggestive of the disease; anti–double-stranded DNA antibody also correlates to the disease; serum creatinine is elevated in lupus; urinalysis; CBC may be as in hemolytic anemia; chest x-ray; head CT scan; brain MRI; electrocardiogram (ECG); cardiac enzymes; and kidney biopsy if diagnosed with lupus nephritis.

Treatment

Topical glucocorticoid for skin manifestations; nonsteroidal antiinflammatory drugs (NSAIDs) for musculoskeletal symptoms; antimalarials such as hydroxychloroquine to treat lupus rashes or joint symptoms and to reduce the incidence of severe disease flares; high-dose methylprednisone intravenously may be given for life- or organ-threatening disease. Patients with lupus must get influenza/pneumococcus vaccine in these immunocompromised patients.

Immunosuppressive agents may be used for severe disease involving kidneys, vasculitis, and central nervous system disease. Secondary infections are promptly treated with antibiotics. With the treatments available today, 10-year survival rates exceed 85%.

Nursing Interventions and Complications

During exacerbations, patients with SLE are very ill and nursing care includes treating the symptoms of any system dysfunction that may be manifested by this disease. The renal and central nervous systems must be assessed, watching for changes in mental status as well as careful intake and output monitoring. Lab values are also monitored by the nurse. Nurses also teach SLE patients and their families about pain management, joint care, signs of infection, resting and conserving energy, and avoiding sunlight. Nursing intervention is also aimed at working with patients emotionally to help them accept the changes and limitations of the disease and coping with a chronic disease. In patients with very severe disease with multiple systems involved and kidney failure, the nurse may support the patient and family through the grieving process preparing for death from the disease.

CLINICAL ALERT

Some people with the disease (SLE) have a virulent course leading to serious impairment of the lungs, heart, brain, or kidney, and the disease may lead to death. In early diagnosis of SLE, death is usually caused by opportunistic organisms and later as the disease attacks the kidney and central nervous system the death rate again is increased. Kidney failure is the most common cause of death in those with lupus. Nurses must closely monitor neurologic and renal systems.

Suggested Readings

Capriotti T, Sheerin S. HAART meds: implications for the older adult patient. *Clin Advisor.* 2012;15(5):23-29.

Corall AH, Mulby AG. *Primary Care Medicine.* 4th ed. Philadelphia, PA: Lippincott Williams & Wilkins; 2000.

Dillon PM. *Nursing Health Assessment: A Critical Thinking, Case Studies Approach.* 2nd ed. Philadelphia, PA: F.A. Davis; 2007.

Domino F. *The 5 Minute Clinical Consults 2011.* 19th ed. Philadelphia, PA: Wolters Kluwer/Lippincott Williams & Wilkins; 2010.

Goroll AH, Mulley AG. *Primary Care Medicine.* 4th ed. Philadelphia, PA: Lippincott Williams & Wilkins; 2000.

Guyton AC, Hall JE. *Textbook of Medical Physiology.* 9th ed. Philadelphia, PA: W.B. Saunders; 1996.

Habif T. *Skin Disease Diagnosis and Treatment.* St. Louis, MO: Mosby; 2001.

Hoppel AM. HIV: still epidemic after 30 years. *Clin Rev.* 2012;22(6):1, 11-13, 33-34.

Kelley WN. *Textbook of Internal Medicine.* 3rd ed. Philadelphia, PA: Lippincott-Raven; 1992.

McPhee SJ, Papadakis MA, Rabow MW. *2011 Current Medical Diagnosis & Treatment.* New York: McGraw-Hill; 2011.

Phipps WJ, Monhahan FD, Sands JK, Marek JF, Neighbors M. *Medical-Surgical Nursing Health and Illness Perspectives.* 7th ed. St Louis, MO: Mosby; 2003.

Robinson M, Cook SS, Currie LM. Systemic lupus erythematosus: a genetic review for advanced practice nurses. *J Am Acad Nurse Pract.* 2011;23(12):629-637.

Taber's Cyclopedic Medical Dictionary. Philadelphia, PA: F.A. Davis; 2009.

Van Leeuwen AM, Poelhuis-Leth DJ. *Davis's Comprehensive Handbook of Laboratory and Diagnostic Tests With Nursing Implications.* 3rd ed. Philadelphia, PA: F.A. Davis; 2009.

Watkins J. Differentiating common bacterial skin infections. *Br J Sch Nurs.* 2012;7(2): 77-78.

Woolliscroft JO. *Handbook of Current Diagnosis & Treatment.* 2nd ed. St. Louis, MO: Mosby; 1998.

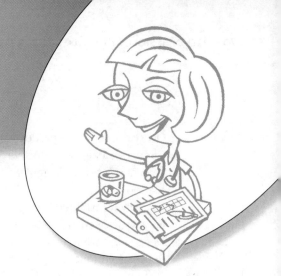

chapter **13**

Reproductive System

LEARNING OBJECTIVES

At the end of this chapter, the reader/student will be able to:

● Describe the physiologic function of the female and male reproductive system

● Discuss the pathologic changes that occur in the female and male reproductive system

● Describe symptoms and diagnostic tests to identify reproductive tract problems

Overview: Female Reproductive System

The principal organs of female reproduction are the ovaries, fallopian tubes, uteruses, and vagina. The development of ova (eggs) occurs in the ovaries and a single ovum is expelled in the middle of each monthly cycle. If the ovum is fertilized, it implants in the uterus, where development of fetus, placenta, and membranes occurs. If the ovum is not fertilized, it is expelled during the menstrual cycle.

The female reproductive system is controlled by hormones. The hypothalamus releases gonadotropin-releasing hormone (GnRH) and stimulates the anterior pituitary to secrete follicle-stimulating hormone (FSH) and luteinizing hormone (LH), and these hormones cause the ovaries to secrete estrogen and progesterone. FSH stimulates follicles to grow in the first part of the menstrual cycle and the estrogen also plays a part, and one dominant follicle remains and LH is then secreted, which is necessary for the final growth of the dominant follicle and in whose ovulation progesterone plays a part. Then, both FSH and LH levels begin to fall as well as estrogen and progesterone, and menstruation occurs. The process occurs approximately every 28 days. If fertilization occurs at ovulation, which is midcycle, then menstruation will not occur. Women can actually get pregnant only about 24 hours a month, which is during ovulation. The normal menstrual cycle is between 21 and 36 days and lasts 3–7 days, with a flow of about 20–80 mL of blood.

Further, estrogen plays a large part in the development of secondary sexual characteristics such as the development of breasts, growth of hair in the pubic area and under the arms, keeps skin soft and smooth, and increases

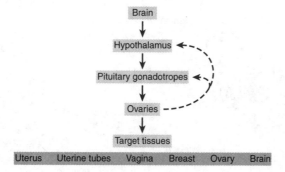

FIGURE 13–1 • Female reproductive neuroendocrine feedback axis. Solid arrows indicate stimulation; dashed arrows indicate inhibition. (Reproduced with permission from McPhee SJ, Hammer GD, eds. *Pathophysiology of Disease: An Introduction to Clinical Medicine.* 6th ed. New York: McGraw-Hill; 2009, figure 22-6.)

the metabolic rate slightly in women. It is important to understand the normal female cycle to better understand the many problems that can occur when the hypothalamus; the pituitary, which release hormones; gonadal (ovary) secretion of estrogen and progesterone; and the uterus do not function exactly as they should (Figure 13–1).

Overview: Male Reproductive System

The male reproductive system consists of testes, where spermatogenesis or the formation of sperm occurs. The sperm empty into the epididymis (a coiled tube) and then lead into the vas deferens, which enlarges to the ampulla of the vas deferens and then into the body of the prostate gland. A seminal vesicle is located on each side of the prostate, and the contents of sperm and seminal fluid pass into an ejaculatory duct leading through the prostate and empty into the urethra, and this semen is ejaculated during the male sexual act through the urethra in the erect penis. Semen is composed of sperm from the testes and fluid from the prostate and a small amount of mucus from another gland. Erection of the penis is caused by parasympathetic impulses from the sacral portion of the spinal cord, and psychological factors also play a part in the male sexual act. The testes (gonads) secrete the hormone testosterone (androgen), which is also responsible for the male secondary sexual characteristic such as hair distribution, deepness of the voice, muscular development, baldness, and increases in the basal metabolic rate.

As with females, the control of sexual functioning begins with GnRH secreted by the hypothalamus and stimulates the anterior pituitary to secrete LH

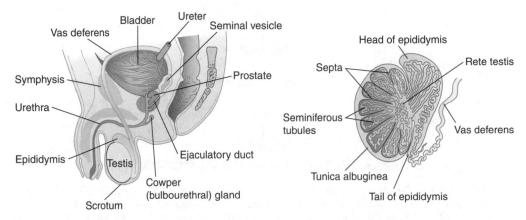

FIGURE 13–2 • Anatomy of male reproductive system (left) and duct system of testis (right). (Reproduced with permission from Ganong WF, ed. *Review of Medical Physiology*. 22nd ed. New York: McGraw-Hill; 2005, figure 23-1.)

and FSH. In males, the LH stimulates the secretion of testosterone and FSH stimulates spermatogenesis (the formation of mature functional sperm) (Figure 13–2).

Women: Menstrual Irregularities

Amenorrhea (absence of a menstrual cycle in the reproductive years) can be either primary or secondary. Primary amenorrhea is when a girl by the age of 16 who has never had a menstrual period. This can be caused by extreme weight gain or loss; eating disorders, excessive exercise; congenital abnormalities; stress; hypothyroidism; hyperprolactinemia (which causes galactorrhea as a result of a pituitary adenoma); imperforate hymen (which would cause obstruction to the normal flow); genetic problem; Cushing disease; ovarian tumor; polycystic ovarian syndrome (discussed later); or pregnancy. Secondary amenorrhea can be caused by disorders of the uterus affecting the outflow, such as destruction of the endometrium as a result of surgery (e.g., dilation and curettage [D&C]) or infections (endometritis); ovarian failure before the age of 40 caused by hypoestrogenism and elevated gonadotropins (FSH, LH) and after the age of 40 would be caused by menopause. Elevated androgens (testosterone, dehydroepiandrosterone sulfate [DHEA-S]) and elevated cortisol levels can alter the normal hormonal menstrual cycle resulting in amenorrhea; and of course the first consideration should be pregnancy or breast-feeding (which needs high prolactin levels to continue). Amenorrhea other than pregnancy or breastfeeding is any condition affecting the normal hormonal menstrual cycle and is called hypothalamic-pituitary-ovarian dysfunction. Depending on the problem, treatment is aimed at treating it. Hyperprolactinemia is treated with bromocriptine.

Another menstrual irregularity is dysmenorrhea, which is very painful menstrual cramps caused by increased prostaglandin production in the endometrium and is often treated with nonsteroidal antiinflammatory drugs (NSAIDs). Fibroids or thickened areas of the endometrium or uterine wall or endometriosis (menstrual implants outside of uterus that cause pain wherever these implants may be) may cause dysmenorrhea. Inflammation and scarring (adhesions) caused by sexually transmitted infections (STI) can result in pelvic inflammation, which causes pain and fever. Some women suffer menstrual migraines that can be incapacitating in the beginning of menstruation.

Dysfunctional uterine bleeding (DUB) is defined as irregular, abnormal bleeding with no definable anatomic abnormality. Menorrhagia is abnormally long, heavy periods. Oligomenorrhea is bleeding that occurs at intervals longer than 35 days. Metrorrhagia is bleeding in between periods. Menometrorrhagia is bleeding that occurs at irregular intervals with heavy flow lasting more than 7 days and polymenorrhea is too frequent periods. DUB can be caused by obesity (fat retains too much estrogen), hormonal imbalance; endometrial polyps or cancer, hypothyroidism or blood dyscrasias or clotting disorders. Abnormal bleeding when there is a positive pregnancy test can be cause by potential loss of the pregnancy.

Clinical Manifestations

Irregular bleeding; painful periods; and in endometriosis pain may be rectal, abdominal, or wherever implants occur; headaches; absence of menstruation; symptoms of endocrine disorders (thyroid, Cushing disease, polycystic ovarian syndrome [PCOS]); and pregnancy symptoms are common.

Diagnostic Tests

Pregnancy test and if positive, sonogram to confirm intrauterine or ectopic; complete blood count (CBC) to assess blood clotting and anemia; prothrombin time (PT); thyroid stimulating hormone (TSH); prolactin level; estrogen and progesterone level; testosterone level; cortisol level; urinalysis; pelvic ultrasound to detect pelvic cysts or masses; FSH/LH levels; possible laparoscopy to diagnose endometriosis or treat pathology; cervical cultures for STIs; erythrocyte sedimentation rate to determine inflammation. GnRH level (to determine hypothalamic function) may indicate the need for rapid treatment for a patient who is hemorrhaging or for women with prolonged heavy menses.

Treatment

Treatment depends on the underlying cause. Irregular bleeding may be treated with hormones such as progesterone, prolactin, or thyroid medication if diagnosed. Surgery may be needed for a dilation and curettage for heavy bleeding or an exploratory laparotomy to determine if there are implants from endometriosis or if fibroids are causing the irregular bleeding. Dysmenorrhea (painful periods) is treated with NSAIDs. Patients with PCOS may be treated with oral contraceptive or metformin.

Nursing Interventions and Complications

Nursing management includes a careful history of menstrual cycle and problems experienced, whether pain or irregular bleeding. Inform the woman on the tests being performed and reason for the tests and educate the woman about the menstrual disorder she has. If the woman has an eating disorder, the nurse does nutritional counseling. The nurse must be alert to pain in pregnancy and the potential for an ectopic pregnancy or loss of pregnancy. Educate the woman that cycles that are irregular with dysfunctional bleeding are usually anovulatory cycles and, if concerned with fertility, refer for treatment of the underlying disorder. Instruct the patient about the medication ordered. Monitor laboratory values. Complication can occur with severe hemorrhage, which may require blood transfusions. Irregular bleeding can also be caused by uterine cancer, ovarian cysts, or ovarian cancer; therefore, appropriate assessment and tests must be done to determine the cause of irregular bleeding.

CLINICAL ALERT

Monitor CBC in women with heavy vaginal bleeding, and those with continued bleeding may require transfusions. If a premenopausal woman does not get regular periods and ultrasonography of the endometrium (lining of the uterus that sheds during menstruation) shows it to be thickened (hyperplasia), there is an increased risk for endometrial cancer.

Menopause

Menopause is defined as the natural cessation of menses for 1 year resulting from estrogen deficiency and not associated with a pathological cause. It is also the end of fertility. In the normal menstrual cycle, the estrogen secreted by the ovarian follicles exerts primarily negative feedback from the dominant follicle to the hypothalamus to continue the normal secretion of hormones for the menstrual cycle, but in menopause when this feedback is absent large quantities of FSH and LH are secreted because the ovaries are not responding. Because the ovaries have failed in menopause, estrogen levels decline as the ovaries account for 90% of the body's production of estrogen. Natural menopause can occur in women older than age 40 years. Actual complete cessation of the menses is usually precipitated by a period called perimenopause where the menstrual cycles become irregular and more and more of the cycles become anovulatory. Many changes occur during menopause as estrogen has many receptors in the body. Many symptoms occur as the woman goes through menopause, including vasomotor symptoms, thinner skin as collagen is lost, visual acuity changes, muscle tone diminishes, and the risk of heart disease becomes equal to heart disease in men. Cardiovascular disease is responsible for more than 50% of the deaths of women in the United States. Bones also start losing density, and risk of fracture increases. There are also estrogen receptors in the external genitalia and loss of the subcutaneous tissue of the labia thins as well as the vagina becomes atrophic, which causes discomfort with sexual intercourse (dyspareunia). Receptors in the brain affected by the loss of estrogen can cause forgetfulness and some mood changes. The management of menopause should be managed individually, and the use of hormone therapy to treat severe symptoms may be an option based on the benefits versus risks. Those who cannot use hormones or chose not to can be treated with selective serotonin reuptake inhibitors (SSRIs), vitamins, or over-the-counter herbal remedies (black cohosh, red clover leaf, soy, valerian root), to treat the hot flashes of menopause.

Clinical Manifestations

Hot flashes; night sweats; anxiety and depression; insomnia; vaginal dryness; fatigue and joint pain; loss of libido (sexual drive); urinary frequency and stress incontinence; heart palpitations; weight gain especially around the midsection; mood changes; and osteopenia/osteoporosis based on bone density test.

Diagnostic Tests

Blood test for FSH >40 mIU/mL and elevated LH; dual-energy x-ray absorptiometry (DEXA) bone scan; and diagnosis is usually made by symptoms and age of the woman. Tests that should be done in women during this period of life are annual mammography; Pap smear; bone density testing; blood work especially for lipids, and if elevated at cardiac workup, TSH and glucose.

Treatment

Hormone therapy treats severe symptoms, but many women cannot take hormones because of risks. Those who cannot or choose not to take hormones can be treated with SSRIs like sertraline HCl (Zoloft) and paroxetine HCl (Paxil), which alleviates the hot flashes. Treatment also includes medications for any abnormal results such as bone density, thyroid disease, high glucose levels, or cardiac problems. Women should exercise regularly to prevent bone loss and heart disease.

Nursing Interventions and Complications

Nurses must counsel women on the risks and benefits to help them to prevent disease and debilitating conditions. Nurses should counsel women to take calcium with vitamin D and extra vitamin D supplementation and to do weight-bearing exercise to preserve bone health. Stress healthy lifestyles and stress management. Advise women to have annual mammographies and perform self breast exams, physical examination annually to monitor blood work and blood pressure, and if smoking to stop but explaining all the risks associated with smoking. Encourage women to exercise at least an hour every day for overall health and well-being. Women during the menopausal and postmenopausal years must be referred for any problems that are cause for concern because cardiovascular risk, osteoporosis, loss of vision, and balance can cause major complications. If the patient is on hormone replacement therapy, many of these risks such as loss of bone and menopausal symptoms and mood changes are relieved.

CLINICAL ALERT

Although menopause is a normal part of the aging woman, heart disease is the number one killer in postmenopausal women. Any cardiac pain or symptoms should be considered an emergency. Nurses caring for women should educate the menopausal woman regarding these risks.

Sexually Transmitted Diseases

There are many sexually transmitted diseases (STDs), some of which can be treated and others such as viral infections that the person has for a lifetime. **Syphilis** is a chronic systemic infection caused by the motile spirochete *Treponema pallidum*. If untreated, it can go through four stages, resulting in death. The rates of syphilis have been decreasing until 2000, when the rate began increasing in men, with men having the disease 6:1 more than women. Although syphilis is treatable, some women at risk such as low socioeconomic status, trading sex for drugs, IV drug abuse, prostitution, and multiple sex partners or no condom use may not seek treatment until they have reached advanced stages. Treatment is with penicillin or other antibiotics. **Gonorrhea** is a bacterial STD that can be symptomatic or asymptomatic in both women and men. In women, gonorrhea infects the cervix and fallopian tubes and is a leading cause of pelvic inflammatory infection. Rectal transmission is through rectal intercourse and it can also be transmitted to infants during birth, causing conjunctivitis and blindness in the infant. The causative agent is *Neisseria gonorrhea*. Some women have mucopurulent cervicitis and a Bartholin abscess as well as having other STDs such as those from infection with chlamydia, trichomonas, monilia, or herpes. Gonorrhea can be treated with ceftriaxone and doxycycline or other combinations. **Chlamydia** is one of the extremely common STDs and like gonorrhea both men and women may be asymptomatic or symptomatic. Men usually have nonspecific urethritis. In women, Chlamydia is associated with cervicitis, salpingitis, and subsequent infertility. *Chlamydia trachomatis* is a parasite that displays some bacterial and some viral qualities. Treatment is with doxycycline or azithromycin. All three syphilis, gonorrhea, and chlamydia are tested in every pregnant woman so that she can be treated and not pass these diseases onto the infant. Syphilis is detected by a blood test, and gonorrhea and chlamydia are tested together through a cervical culture. **Trichomoniasis** is a flagellated anaerobic protozoan. The organism lives in the vagina and urethra of women and the urethra in men; therefore, it is transmitted during vaginal-penile intercourse. The symptoms are a foul smelling, yellow-green, frothy vaginal discharge. Women may report dyspareunia (painful intercourse) and dysuria. Men may have urethritis or prostatitis. Trichomoniasis is diagnosed by a culture taken because of symptoms, and treatment is with metronidazole. **Bacterial vaginosis** is a form of vaginitis most prevalent among childbearing women. The causative organism is *Gardnerella vaginalis* (diagnosed by a culture) and results from disruption of the homeostatic state of the vagina. Bacterial vaginosis can result in preterm labor, chorioamnionitis (infection in the membranes around the fetus). Women may be asymptomatic or complain of a malodorous vaginal discharge. The Ph of the discharge is greater than 4.5 and a culture is used to diagnose bacterial vaginosis. Treatment is metronidazole vaginal gel or orally, or clindamycin vaginal or oral. **Candidiasis** is a common cause of vaginitis caused by *Candida albicans*. It is caused by an upset in the homeostatic balance of the vagina, which leads to an overgrowth of the organism. The recent use of antibiotics, diabetes, or pregnancy can predispose the woman to have candidiasis. The symptoms are vaginal itching, burning, and irritation with vaginal discharge, which is usually thick and white. If this is transmitted to the neonate during delivery, the infant develops an oral infection called thrush. A vaginal culture or a wet mount viewing under a microscope will diagnose candidiasis. Treatment is clotrimazole or terconazole vaginal cream or fluconazole tablet. **Herpes simplex virus (HSV-2)** is a viral STD that produces genital lesions after direct contact with an infected individual. The lesions can be very painful and there is no cure for this viral disease. Men and women are affected. If a pregnant woman has an outbreak of lesions before delivery and delivers vaginally, the neonate can contract the virus and an infection of the central nervous symptom may develop and morbidity and mortality may occur. The primary outbreak of herpes causes very painful ulcer-like sores, chills, fever, and malaise, but recurrent bouts of HSV are not as severe although the sores are still painful. A viral culture of one of the open lesions confirms the virus. Treatment is with one of the antivirals such as acyclovir (Zovirax) or famciclovir (Famvir) for acute attacks and daily thereafter to suppress the attacks. The virus is always present and can still be transmitted to others if condoms are not used. **Condylomata acuminata** is caused by the human papilloma virus (HPV) types 6, 11, 16, 18, 31, and 33 and produces soft, skin-colored, fleshy warts that appear on the vagina, cervix, around the external genitalia, and the rectum. Once HPV is contracted, there is little that can be done as it is a virus. There is a vaccine that consists of three injections within 6 months that will prevent the virus if the vaccine is received prior to sexual intercourse or contracting the virus. Today, it is the most common sexually transmitted viral disease and spreads very easily. HPV on the cervix must be monitored by frequent Pap smears and by colposcopic tests to monitor the virus, as HPV is the cause of cervical cancer. External warts can be treated with acid to remove them or with a cream to use at home (Aldara [imiquimod]). If many external warts are present, removal with laser may be required. Abnormal Pap test or the presence of HPV on the Pap result requires investigation of the cervix by colposcopy and if the lesion is of a high grade, laser is used on the cervix to remove some of the

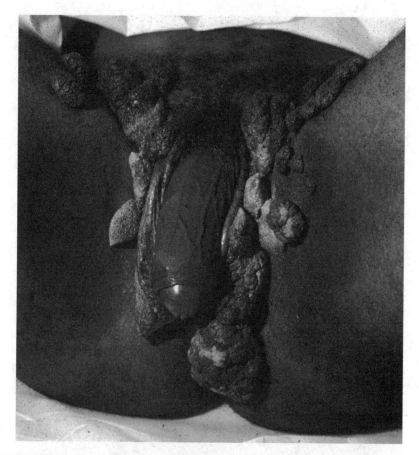

FIGURE 13–3 • Giant condylomata acuminata in a man with AIDS. (Reproduced with permission from Usatine RP, et al. *The Color Atlas of Family Medicine.* New York: McGraw-Hill; 2009, figure 127-10. Courtesy of Jack Resneck, Sr.)

virus, and frequent monitoring is required. If there are any cancer cells detected, a hysterectomy is done to avoid cervical cancer spreading (Figures 13–3 and 13–4).

Clinical Manifestations

Lesions (sores or warts) on the genital area, vaginal discharge, pain in the pelvic area, burning or itching inside the vagina or in the genital area, foul-smelling greenish discharge, painful genital ulcer-like sores, and swollen abscesses in the Bartholin gland.

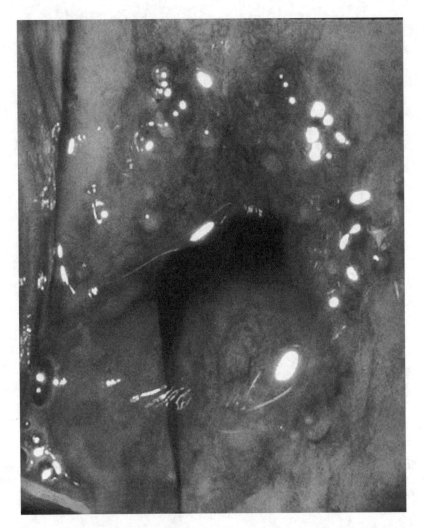

FIGURE 13–4 • Chlamydial cervicitis with ectopy, mucoid discharge, and bleeding. The cervix is inflamed and friable. (Reproduced with permission from Usatine RP, et al. *The Color Atlas of Family Medicine*. New York: McGraw-Hill; 2009, figure 81-1. Courtesy of Connie Celum and Walter Stamm, Seattle STD/HIV Prevention Training Center.)

Diagnostic Tests

Syphilis blood test for Rapid Plasma Reagin (RPR) or Venereal Disease Research Laboratory (VDRL), the fluorescent treponemal antibody-absorption test (FTA-ABS; confirms after RPR or VDRL is positive), HSV viral culture of open sore or type-specific serologic, Western blot, gonorrhea caused by *N gonorrhoeae* (GC)/chlamydia culture, vaginal culture (e.g., AFFIRM test for candidiasis, bacterial vaginosis, and trichomonas), Pap with HPV; if HPV found on cervix, perform colposcopy with biopsy, and pelvic sonogram if pelvic pain present.

Treatment

Treatment is based on the diagnosis. Candidiasis is treated with terconazole (Terazol) or miconazole nitrate (Monistat) creams; herpes is treated with antiviral medications such as valacyclovir HCl (Valtrex) or famciclovir; bacterial vaginosis is treated with metronidazole (MetroGel); chlamydia is treated with azithromycin; gonorrhea is treated with ceftriaxone or azithromycin and partner needs treatment also; syphilis is treated with intramuscular penicillin and partner needs treatment also. HPV has no treatment and the cervix needs close monitoring, and cervical changes diagnosed during colposcopy may require laser surgery or conization (removal of diseased part of cervix). External warts (condyloma) can be removed by acid, laser, cryosurgery (liquid nitrogen), or by use of a medication called Aldara (imiquimod).

Nursing Interventions and Complications

Nurses should assess adolescent sexual behavior and counsel on the risks of unprotected sex. Encourage clients to complete all medication prescribed for STIs. Educate and reinforce the need to have partner always use latex condoms. Patients with frequent candidiasis infection should be instructed to avoid tight-fitting pants, wear cotton underwear, take showers not baths, and avoid bubble bath and bath gels. For very frequent yeast infections, patients should be screened for glucose levels as yeast infections are frequent in diabetics. If infection can be treated, instruct the patient on use of medication and teach prevention to avoid STIs in the future. If the client does not have HPV encourage the vaccine (Gardasil) that prevents HPV, and if the client has HPV explain the reason for frequent testing and Pap tests. Instruct the client not to have sex until both the client and the partner are treated in infections such as gonorrhea, syphilis, and chlamydia. The nurse should assess risk factors in the client's life that would make them at risk for certain STDs and test for them.

CLINICAL ALERT

The complications of STDs such as untreated syphilis can lead to neurologic problems and death, and untreated gonorrhea or chlamydia can cause pelvic inflammatory disease, causing infertility due to scarred fallopian tubes, and HPV can cause cervical cancer.

Polycystic Ovarian Syndrome

This is a multilevel abnormality characterized by ovarian dysfunction, with oligomenorrhea, chronic anovulation, infertility, androgen excess with hirsutism (excessive hair growth), and acne. The condition often starts at puberty and is associated with obesity, hypertension, diabetes, metabolic syndrome, hyperlipidemia, infertility, and insulin resistance syndrome. Affected women have elevated levels of LH, which cause stimulation of the theca (sheath) in small ovarian follicles to secrete large amounts of androstenedione (precursor to testosterone) and testosterone. For reasons that are not understood completely, follicular growth is abnormal and no prominent follicle develops; therefore, there is no normal LH surge triggered midcycle, which results in no ovulation and no menses. In PCOS, androgen excess is the core defect. Increased androgen levels produced by the ovaries, and small amounts from the adrenal and peripheral adipose tissue, interfere with the normal hypothalamic sensitivity to negative feedback of the ovary, which causes normal secretion of hormones in response to the estrogen and progesterone from the ovaries. PCOS causes increased secretion of GnRH, to a level that favors increased LH secretion, which stimulates the ovaries to continue to produce more androgens. There is a decrease in the FSH level, which impairs follicle development, leading to prolonged periods of oligomenorrhea (no menses). There are also some metabolic changes that occur with PCOS such as insulin resistance and hyperinsulinemia. Together with the free androgen levels and the insulin resistance, there is the release of fatty acids from the liver and adipose tissue, which contributes to the dyslipidemia that is associated with PCOS. Thus, PCOS is recognized as the most common endocrinopathy in reproductive-age women and affects approximately 5%–10% of women. Abdominal obesity is common and metabolic dysfunction is greater in adolescents with PCOS. Young women may have a hard time coping with this syndrome, and become depressed because of the effect on their reproductive endocrine/metabolic and skin systems. Endometrial hyperplasia caused by no menses and high levels of estrogen levels must be managed, as it can lead to endometrial cancer. If the patient wants to become pregnant, ovulation induction can be tried with clomiphene citrate (Clomid), and sometimes treatment with metformin can result in ovulation and so metformin is often used throughout the pregnancy (Figure 13–5).

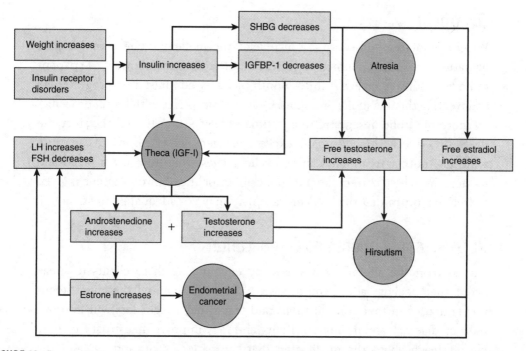

FIGURE 13–5 • Pathogenesis of the various clinical manifestations of the polycystic ovary syndrome. SHBG, steroid hormone-binding globulin; IGFBP-1, insulin-like growth factor binding protein-1; IGF, insulin-like growth factor; FSH, follicle-stimulating hormone; LH, luteinizing hormone. (Redrawn, with permission, from Barnes HV. *Clinical Medicine: Selected Problems with Pathophysiologic Correlations.* Year Book Medical Publishers; 1988.)

Clinical Manifestations

Obesity; hirsutism (hair may be on chin, all over face, chest, upper legs); facial acne; anovulation; amenorrhea; infertility; insulin resistance; obstructive sleep apnea; and hypertension. There may be a thickened endometrium (lining of the uterus) that may lead to endometrial cancer. This must be carefully monitored by ultrasonographs to assess endometrial thickness.

Diagnostic Tests

Testosterone and DHEA-S level; LH/FSH (if LH is >2.5%, 50% will have PCOS); estrogen levels are increased; glucose and insulin level; transvaginal sonogram (enlarged ovaries with small follicles); sex hormone–binding globulin (SHBG) is decreased; lipid profile.

Treatment

Weight reduction and exercise can reverse the metabolic effects and induce ovulation. Treatment is aimed at decreasing the androgens, allowing the patient to have a monthly or every-third-month bleed by administering progesterone and treating the metabolic problems. Oral contraceptives with low androgenicity (norethindrone, desogestrel, norgestimate) may be beneficial as they increase the SHBG levels, which decreases excess androgens and estrogen and can cause a bleed. Another treatment can be cyclic progesterone to cause a bleed and metformin to help correct the metabolic abnormalities. Spironolactone is given to treat hirsutism that the oral contraceptive may not adequately treat.

Nursing Interventions and Complications

Nurses treat the altered body image by encouraging these clients to speak about their feelings about the disease. Nurses also counsel the client about prevention of further complications and teach that weight loss will improve their cardiac risk and insulin sensitivity and may improve menstrual function. Nurses teach about the medication that the patient takes and explains the ordered tests to the patient. The complications that can occur as a result of PCOS is diabetes mellitus, breast cancer, and endometrial carcinoma due to high estrogen levels. These patients need to be treated and observed frequently to avoid these potential complications.

> ### CLINICAL ALERT
>
> The high levels of estrogen in PCOS patients with no menses leads to a build-up of the endometrial lining that leads to endometrial cancer and has a relationship to an increase in breast cancer. The patients also have increased lipids and obesity, which put them at a greater risk for cardiac problems. Patients must be treated to have a bleed at least every 3 months. Emotional support is indicated for these patients who have infertility, obesity, and all the symptoms as well as many risks.

Deep Vein Thrombosis

Thrombi develop from platelets, fibrin, and both red and white cells. They can develop as either a single or multiple clots within the deep veins of the extremities or pelvis, usually accompanied by inflammation of the vessel wall.

Most deep vein thromboses (DVTs) develop in the pelvis or lower extremities, but they can develop in the vessels of the upper extremities, leading to the heart. Approximately 2 million Americans are diagnosed with DVT each year and at least half of these diagnosed will develop a pulmonary emboli. The lungs are rich in heparin and plasma activators and can effectively dissolve some thrombi. But if the thrombi are too large it can lodge in an artery and occlude perfusion to the lung, which can be fatal. The causes of DVT are situations that cause hypercoagulability, damage to the vessel wall, or venous stasis, and these three factors are called Virchow triad. DVT involves the partial or complete blockage of a vein by a clot, which is the cause of significant morbidity and mortality. Surgery is a major risk especially pelvic surgery in women. DVTs occur more commonly in women including during pregnancy. Immobility caused by surgery, paralysis, casting or traction, prolonged travel, aging, sedentary lifestyle, and inherited coagulation defects can all cause DVT. In women, estrogen is thrombogenic (capable of producing blood clots); therefore, pregnancy, use of oral contraceptives, hormone replacement therapy, and obesity can increase the chance of a woman developing a DVT. It is now recommended by the College of Obstetricians and Gynecologists that pharmacologic thromboprophylaxis (use of an anticoagulant such as a low-molecular-weight heparin, e.g., Luvenox or Fragmin) begin 2 hours prior to gynecologic surgery.

Clinical Manifestations

Pain and tenderness in the affected area; unilateral edema or swelling in the affected leg or extremity; redness and warmth if phlebitis (inflammation of the vein) is extensive and can be palpated like a firm vessel; fever; and positive Homan sign (calf tenderness when the foot of the affected leg is dorsiflexed) are commonly found. If the clot has traveled to the lung, pain and difficulty breathing is apparent, and if the clot is in the heart, sudden chest pain and depending on vessel occluded can result in a heart attack or death.

Diagnostic Tests

D-dimer test (assists in detection of DVT); CBC with platelets, activated partial thromboplastin (aPTT) and prothrombin time (PT) and International Normalized Ratio (INR); arterial blood gases (ABGs); chest x-ray; electrocardiograph (ECG); ultrasonography with color Doppler is in the extremity; contrast venography; magnetic resonance imaging (MRI).

Treatment

Treatment is aimed at preventing a pulmonary embolism by treating the DVT and includes heparin, and thrombolytic therapy such as streptokinase, urokinase, or tissue plasminogen activator (tPA). Sometimes, the diagnosis of DVT is missed as 80% are asymptomatic until severe symptoms arise. If the circulation of an extremity is compromised, a surgical removal of the thrombus may be required (thrombectomy), or a filter is placed in the vena cava to trap the clot before it travels to the lung or heart (Greenfield filter).

Nursing Interventions and Complications

Nursing diagnosis includes ineffective tissue perfusion and monitors the perfusion of the affected leg, including neurovascular assessment noting the pain, swelling, temperature of area, and circumference of the affected leg versus the unaffected one, and take pulses to determine if there is an occlusion. Acute pain will be managed with medication and positioning to decrease edema. The nurse also assesses the patient for acute complications of a clot that has dislodged from a peripheral vein to the lungs or heart. The nurse will also prevent DVT through the knowledge of what causes DVT and early ambulation of surgical patients, apply compression stockings, and check the Homan sign. In addition, the nurse will educate clients on the risk of developing DVT such as prolonged sitting, medications such as oral contraceptives, and hormone replacement therapy.

CLINICAL ALERT

Complication of a DVT can be a pulmonary embolism or an embolism that travels to the heart and both of these can be fatal, if not diagnosed rapidly and effectively treated.

Pregnancy-Induced Hypertension

This is now referred to as **Gestational Hypertension**. Toxemia was a previous term used but there are no toxins in gestational hypertension. Every day in the United States, 1,000 pregnant women will learn they have high blood pressure. Gestational hypertension is hypertension that occurs after 20 weeks' gestation without proteinuria, and a return to normal pregnancy after delivery. The pathophysiology of gestational hypertension is unknown although many theories exist none can explain the widespread pathologic changes that occur. Generalized vasospasm results in the high blood pressure and reduces the blood supply to the brain, liver, kidneys, placenta, and lungs. Gestational hypertension is diagnosed when a blood pressure of 140/90 or higher is reached on more than two occasions at least 6 hours apart. Gestational hypertension is different than chronic hypertension, as chronic hypertension appears before the 20th week or is hypertension that occurs before the current pregnancy and continues after birth. Gestational hypertension is the second leading cause of maternal death in the United States, the first being an embolism. Hypertension is the most common cause of complications in pregnancy and occurs in 12%–20% of pregnancies. The vasospasm that occurs in hypertension, decreases liver perfusion causes liver dysfunction and a subcapsular hemorrhage. This causes epigastric pain and elevated liver enzymes. Decreased brain perfusion leads to small hemorrhage of the brain, causing headache, blurred vision, and hyperactive deep tendon reflexes. An imbalance in clotting factors leads to an increase in thromboxane (a potent vasoconstrictor), resulting in a stimulation of platelet aggregation, which adds to the hypertensive state. Decreased perfusion to the kidneys reduces the glomerular filtration rate (GFR) and the output decreases; the BUN and creatinine increase and edema from the capillary permeability increases; and protein is spilled into the urine. Treatment depends on the severity of the disease. In mild preeclampsia, a woman may be sent home on bed rest and to remain in a lateral position to improve circulation to the baby. Blood pressure is monitored frequently and any change requires hospitalization. Any woman with severe preeclampsia requires complete rest and a quiet dark room to reduce any stimulus. Sedatives may be ordered and seizure precautions instituted. Severe preeclampsia may progress to HELLP syndrome, where hemolysis (H) (destruction of red blood cells), the elevated liver enzymes (EL), and low platelet count (LP). The physiology of HELLP is that hemolysis occurs when the red blood cells become fragmented as they pass through the damaged blood vessels and elevated liver enzymes occur because of reduced blood flow to the liver due to obstruction with fibrin deposits. Low platelets result from vascular damage causing vasospasm and platelets aggregate at the damaged area. This is a serious complication, and the mother could develop a liver hematoma or liver rupture, a stroke, cardiac arrest, pulmonary edema, renal damage, hypoxic encephalopathy, and maternal or neonatal death. Depending on the age of the fetus, delivery is the best treatment and maternal risk versus the life of the infant complicates this potentially lethal pregnancy-related condition.

Clinical Manifestations

Hypertension, headache, visual disturbances, dizziness, generalized edema, oliguria, epigastric or right upper quadrant pain, hyperactive deep tendon reflexes, pulmonary edema, confusion, seizures, and nausea.

Diagnostic Tests

Check urine for proteinuria, monitor laboratory results for liver and renal problems, CBC with platelets, coagulation profile, 24-hour urine for protein and creatinine, monitor daily kick count of the baby, and have a non-stress test (NST) weekly, ultrasonography to measure growth of baby and cord, placenta functioning, and amniotic fluid index. If seizure occurs, get computed tomographic (CT) scan and MRI.

Treatment

Treatment includes magnesium sulfate to prevent seizures, antihypertensives, diuretics, and correction of the coagulopathies such as packed red cells, fresh-frozen plasma, or platelets.

Nursing Interventions and Complications

Nursing management is to obtain good health history and provide close monitoring of the mother and the fetus. Monitor blood pressure, symptoms, and laboratory values to determine if the client is going into HELLP syndrome. Maintain the women in the lateral position (to provide best oxygenation for the fetus) in a dark, quiet environment and cluster assessments to let the mother rest. Monitor medications such as magnesium sulfate by observing the neurologic status. Explain all medication and tests to the patient. Observe for signs of cerebral irritation or signs of a seizure. Encourage the patient to drink water for mild preeclampsia. Suction and administer oxygen as needed in severe preeclampsia. Close monitoring of intake and output.

CLINICAL ALERT

The complications of severe preeclampsia with HELLP syndrome are pulmonary edema, maternal liver or renal failure, abruptio placentae, fetal demise, and maternal death. The nurse must closely monitor the patient and seek immediate help for any change. The best treatment is delivery of the fetus, and depending on the age may pose decisions as to the life of infant or mother. Nurses are involved in the discussion regarding these ethical dilemmas and the family wishes.

Disseminated Intravascular Coagulation

Disseminated intravascular coagulation (DIC) is an acquired syndrome characterized by diffuse intravascular activation of coagulation arising from different causes. It is a bleeding disorder and affected individuals can experience widespread external and internal bleeding and clotting. With DIC, the anticoagulation and procoagulation factors are activated at the same time that thromboplastin (a clotting factor) is released into the maternal circulation as a result of complications such as abruptio placentae, which result in clot formation. Circulating levels of prothrombin activate widespread clotting throughout the microcirculation. This consumes and uses up other clotting factors such as fibrinogen and platelets. The entire fibrinolytic system tries to destroy the clot and as a result, there is a decrease in clotting factors and an increase in circulating anticoagulants, leaving the person's blood unable to clot. The lab results show low hemoglobin, hematocrit, platelets, and fibrinogen and elevated levels of fibrin split products (material released in the bloodstream when fibrin in a blood clot is digested by plasmin). The causes of DIC are abruptio placentae, dead fetus retention, infection (gram-negative organisms), malignancy, trauma, missed abortion, amniotic fluid embolism, and eclampsia. Treatment of DIC is to treat the underlying condition that caused the DIC with fluid and replace clotting factors. When abruptio placentae has caused the DIC, delivery of the fetus and placenta must be done to stop the production of thromboplastin. This is accomplished by giving heparin intravenously to stop the clotting cascade. The heparin is given carefully close to the time of birth to decrease the change of a postpartum hemorrhage. After the heparin therapy is completed, blood and platelets can be administered. In some facilities, antithrombin III factor, fibrinogen, or cryoprecipitate may be given. As DIC progresses, there is bleeding of the mucous membranes and tissues, which appear as petechiae and ecchymoses, and oral, gastrointestinal, and rectal bleeding. The patient may be hypoxic, hypotensive, and acidotic. DIC patients are gravely ill and can bleed from several sites.

Clinical Manifestations

Skin: petechiae, purpura, ecchymosis, oozing from venipuncture sites, or wounds. Renal: hematuria, oliguria, and uremia. Respiratory: epistaxis, pulmonary hemorrhage, and hypoxemia. Neurologic: convulsions, delirium, and coma.

Diagnostic Tests

D-dimer is positive in DIC, PTT is increased, thrombocytes are low, PT is increased, fibrinogen is low, increased fibrin split products, decreased anti-thrombin III, if infection is thought to be the cause, get a blood culture.

Treatment

The underlying causative disorder must be treated with either antimicrobials if infection, chemotherapy, surgery, or delivery of fetus. Blood products such as platelets and fresh-frozen plasma are given if there is significant hemorrhage. In cases of continued bleeding, treatment with heparin is used to inhibit the underlying thrombotic process.

Nursing Interventions and Complications

Fluid body deficit is met by assessing every area for bleeding. Nurses monitor the blood work and patients with DIC are usually treated in the intensive care unit because of the close monitoring required. Nurses also provide emotional support to the patient and the family, who are fearful that the patient may die. Monitor intake and output carefully. Assess the patient for any signs of organ and respiratory failure. Nurses should know the many potential causes of DIC and assess those at high risk for the development of symptoms so that the underlying condition can be treated before DIC becomes critical.

> **CLINICAL ALERT**
>
> *DIC can result in renal failure, respiratory distress, and neurologic changes. If DIC is caused by an infection, septic shock and the circulating toxins from the bacteria activate the clotting mechanism and plug the vessels, thereby diminishing the delivery of oxygen and nutrients, which further exacerbates the shock. Septic shock can cause death in 85% of patients. Nurses must carefully assess patient with risk for DIC and patients diagnosed with gram-negative organisms should be a priority because of the risk for death with DIC.*

Premenstrual Syndrome and Premenstrual Dysphoric Disorder

Premenstrual syndrome (PMS) describes a wide range of symptoms that occur usually 1–2 weeks prior to menses. The symptoms usually interfere with some aspect of life. It is estimated that approximately 80% of all women experience some combination of emotional, physical, or behavioral symptoms. PMS usually occurs in the luteal phase or last half of the menstrual cycle. The exact cause of PMS is unknown but it may be related to interaction between cyclic hormonal changes and neurotransmitters such as serotonin. **Premenstrual dysphoric mood disorder (PMDD)** is a more severe form of PMS. An imbalance of the hormones estrogen and progesterone may contribute to the severe symptoms of PMDD. It is listed in the *Diagnostic and Statistical Manual of Mental Disorders, Fourth Edition (DSM IV)*. Treatment may include oral contraception to stop the normal hormonal changes, diuretics, antidepressants, analgesics, and some comfort measures such as heat application or warm baths. Exercise can help with symptoms, and eliminating caffeine, soda, chocolate, fat, processed foods, and alcohol during the premenstrual phase may help. Taking a good multivitamin with B vitamins may also help.

Clinical Manifestations

In **PMS**, irritability, depression, fatigue, headache, abdominal bloating, breast tenderness, weight gain, and sleep disturbance. Feeling overwhelmed with normal stressors, and food cravings for salty and sweet foods. In **PMDD**, more severe symptoms such as severe depression, feeling of inadequacy, anxiety, severe mood swings, decreased interest in activities usually enjoyed, difficulty concentrating, fatigue, appetite changes, breast tenderness or swelling, headaches, and joint and muscle pain. These symptoms can impact the ability to conduct usual activities such as work or going to school.

Diagnostic Tests

Symptoms occur usually 1 week prior to menses and end shortly after menses begin. Other tests involve examining TSH levels to rule out thyroid disease and levels of 25-OH vitamin D to determine if vitamin D supplementation may help.

Treatment

SSRIs for mood, alprazolam (during the luteal phase), danazol, spironolactone to reduce fluid retention, calcium carbonate, vitamin B_6, or oral contraceptives can be used. Reduce salt, sugar, caffeine, and alcohol.

Nursing Interventions and Complications

Office nurses must be aware of the severity of especially PMDD symptoms and when a patient calls with emotional complaints during the premenstrual phase, the patient should be seen right away and treatment begun. Nurses should assess patients for symptoms occurring prior to the patient's menses to assess the severity and the need for treatment. Patients with PMDD have mood swings and depression, and during the period when the woman is feeling out of control suicide risk needs to be assessed closely by the nurse and immediate referral made.

> ### CLINICAL ALERT
>
> *Patients who suffer from severe PMDD feel overwhelmed, and the disorder can greatly affect their daily life. These patients should be treated. These are not life-threatening disorders.*

Male: Benign Prostatic Hyperplasia

The prostate gland lies just under the bladder in the pelvis and surrounds the midportion of the urethra in men. It is usually small, about the size of a walnut, and enlarges with age. The purpose of the prostate and the seminal vesicles above it is to produce the fluid that nourishes the sperm and produces most of the volume of fluid that is ejaculated. Enlargement of the prostate gland can cause significant urinary problems because of its location under the bladder. The exact cause of prostate enlargement is not known, but as a man ages the amount of testosterone decreases and the amount of estrogen increase. There is cell proliferation, causing the prostate to enlarge and change consistency. Parts of the gland enlarge, whereas other parts become nodular. When this occurs, it impinges on the urethra and the urethra elongates and compresses the flow of urine. Urinary retention caused by the hypertrophy of the prostate can lead to high bladder pressure, leading to kidney problems. This is a benign condition and occurs in approximately 50% of men older than age 50 years and 75% of men older than age 70 years. At first, certain medications may be tried such as tamsulosin HCl (Flomax) or finasteride (Proscar). For patients who have recurrent problems such as obstruction of urine, with frequent urinary infections, surgical intervention may be indicated. The surgery is called a transurethral prostatectomy (TURP). This surgery is done through the urethra using a resectoscope that cuts and cauterizes the tissue. A Foley catheter is inserted and frequent bladder irrigations are necessary to remove the blood and prevent excessive clotting or clot retention. As a result of this surgery, orgasms may be affected and a small number of men may become incontinent.

Clinical Manifestations

Urinary frequency, nocturia, weak urinary stream, hesitancy (difficulty initiating urination), feeling of incomplete emptying, urgency, gross hematuria, urine dribbling.

Diagnostic Tests

Pressure flow studies, cystoscopy, biopsy to rule out malignancy of the prostate, abdominal sonogram, PSA lab test, urinalysis and culture and sensitivity, BUN, and creatinine test, and digital examination to determine the size of the prostate.

Treatment

Medications to increase urinary flow such as terazosin (Hytrin) and tamsulosin. If not, urinary catheterization or TURP.

Nursing Interventions and Complications

Prior to surgery, nurses must take a thorough history and make a list of medications used, especially ones that could cause bleeding such as ASA (Aspirin; acetylsalicylic acid) or NSAIDs. The nurse assesses the patient's understanding of the surgery and explains the three-way Foley that will allow the nurse to irrigate the surgical site to preventing clot formation. Encourage fluid intake and after Foley is taken out, monitor for signs of infection and provide pain control. Encourage verbalization about fears about sexual functioning and coping skills. The patient is told to avoid alcohol.

CLINICAL ALERT

Complications of BPH are urinary retention (acute or chronic), bladder stones, prostatitis, renal failure, and loss of blood with hematuria.

Erectile Dysfunction

Another word for erectile dysfunction is impotence. This is a man's inability to attain a penile erection sufficient to complete sexual intercourse. Normal penile erection required full functioning of the vascular, nervous, and hormonal systems. Erectile dysfunction (ED) is low in men less than 40 years of age but increases with age. The causes can be multifactorial and some psychological reasons may be stress, anxiety, or depression. Medical reasons for ED can be vascular, such as cardiovascular disease, diabetes, benign prostatic hyperplasia, certain medications (antihypertensives), neurologic disorders, substance abuse, and smoking. One in 10 men in the United States has chronic ED, and 46.6% of men aged 50–69 years have ED. In ED, the blood volume in the erectile chambers of corpora cavernosa is inadequate to dilate the arteries in the penis. ED in men can cause anxiety, depression, guilt, feelings of inadequacy, and relationship issues. Treatments range from medications such as sildenafil (Viragr) or tadalafil (Cialis) to testosterone replacement, surgical implantation of a penile prosthesis, vacuum erectile pump, or penile injections.

Clinical Manifestations

Inability to maintain an erection, inability to achieve an erection, reduced body hair, peripheral vascular disease, or emotional disorders are most common.

Diagnostic Tests

Dorsal nerve somatosensory-evoked potentials, 24-hour zinc level, penile-brachial blood pressure, aortogram, dynamic cavernosography, penile blood pressure, testosterone level, lipid profile and prostate-specific antigen (PSA), glucose level, TSH, and psychological testing.

Treatment

Medications used to increase erection are sildenafil, vardenafil HCl (Levitra), and tadalafil (Cialis). If these do not work, penile injections with alprostadil, which causes smooth muscle relaxation of the arterial blood vessels, and testosterone supplementation is also used. A surgical implantation of a penile prosthesis can be done if the above treatments fail. A complementary treatment is Yohimbine.

Nursing Interventions and Complications

The nursing diagnosis of sexual dysfunction and anxiety are treated by the nurse providing emotional support and explaining alternative methods for intimacy that will provide a positive sexual interaction. Support the man when surgical intervention is what the man chooses. Explain contraindications to taking medications to attain an erection such as taking nitrates for heart problems or hypotensive medications. Explain the side effects of taking the oral medications such as flushing, headache, dizziness, hypotension, and vision changes.

CLINICAL ALERT

Men taking more than the required dose or those who take medications to enhance a normal erection may suffer priapism or a prolonged painful erection that may require going to the emergency room for treatment to relax the penis. Men taking nitrates and certain heart medications can suffer a severe potentially lethal hypotensive crisis if they take medications to enhance erection. Nurses need to teach the patients about the medications and side effects and the life-threatening risks of taking these medications with other heart medications. The patients should be instructed to see their health care providers to discuss the risks.

Inflammatory Disorders: Urethritis

Urethral inflammation marked by painful urination, pruritis, hematuria, and/or discharge. It is usually a result of an STI and less commonly caused by an autoimmune disorder, trauma, or chemical irritation. The predominant age of young men with urethritis is between 15 and 24 years, which correlates with sexual activity.

Epididymitis

Inflammation of the oblong organ resting on and beside the posterior surface of the testicles. It is a secretory duct in each testicle. In acute epididymitis, pain can last for up to 6 weeks and chronic epididymitis can last greater than 3 months. There is scrotal pain and swelling and there can be induration and eventual scrotal wall edema. There is pain, redness, and swelling, and fever and chills are common. The man with epididymitis walks with a waddling gait to protect the groin and scrotum. This can be caused by an ascending infection via the ejaculatory duct through the vas deferens into the epididymis. This is the most common intrascrotal inflammation in adult males. Infection usually results in three ways: (1) from infection introduced during a surgical or diagnostic procedure, (2) organism such as *Escherichia coli* or in some cases structural abnormalities, and (3) sexually transmitted organisms such as *C. trachomatis* and *N. gonorrhoeae*. Some risk factors are urethral or meatal stricture; surgical procedures; high-risk sexual behavior; anal intercourse; presence of foreskin; prolonged sedentary periods; constipation and HIV-immunosuppressed patients. Treatment is antibiotics.

Orchitis

Inflammation or infection of the testicle. This may be caused by pyogenic bacteria, gonococci, tubercle bacilli, or viruses (e.g., paramyxovirus responsible for mumps) or it may follow any septicemia. Orchitis can often occur after epididymitis. A collection of fluid in the testes called a hydrocele occurs. The signs and symptoms are similar to epididymitis; however, in orchitis it is systemic instead of localized. The systemic effect may produce nausea, vomiting, and severe pain radiating to the inguinal canal. Fibrosis of the testicle can occur and atrophy of the testes occurs in 20%–30% of patients, and sterility occurs in about 20% of cases. If the other testis is not involved, fertility is still intact. Treatment is antibiotics and medication to reduce the pain and swelling.

Any postpubertal boy or man who is exposed to mumps may be given gamma-globulin as mumps causes infertility in men. To determine the man is infertile, a sperm analysis would be done (Figure 13–6).

Prostatitis

Inflammation or very painful condition affecting the prostate gland usually as a result of an infection. In general, the prostate gland surrounds the neck of the bladder and the urethra and secretes slightly alkaline fluid that forms the seminal fluid or ejaculate. There are about 2 million cases annually in the United States and the predominant age is between 30 and 50 years.

Bacterial prostatitis occurs more frequently in patients with HIV. An acute infection causes fever, perineal pain, dysuria, and obstructive symptoms. Risk

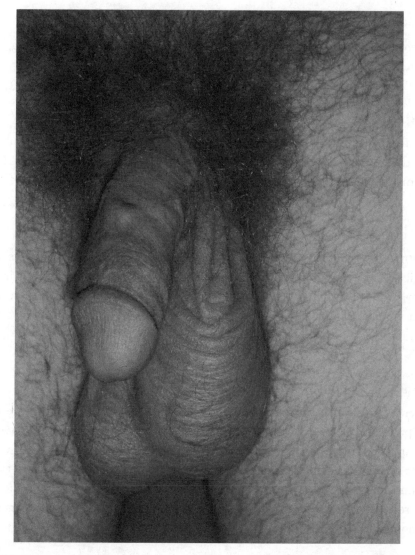

FIGURE 13–6 • **Orchitis.** Unilateral testicular pain, swelling, scrotal erythema, and edema is seen in this patient with parotitis. (Reproduced with permission from Knoop K, et al. *Atlas of Emergency Medicine.* 3rd ed. New York: McGraw-Hill; 2009, figure 8-7. Photo contributor: Alan B. Storrow, MD.)

factors are prostatic calculi, urinary tract infection, trauma such as horseback riding, sexual abstinence, urethral stricture, and surgery on the prostate (TURP). Treatment includes antibiotics, depending on the organism found and if prostatitis is acute or chronic, and pain management. The causes can be many different organisms.

Clinical Manifestations

Severe tenderness and pain in the area involved, fever, dysuria, swelling, and urethral discharge (in epididymitis and prostatitis).

Diagnostic Tests

Urinalysis, urine culture and sensitivity, ultrasound, gram staining on all culture of either semen, expressed prostate, or urethral secretions, CBC, gonorrhea/chlamydia testing on sample.

Treatment

Treatment is antibiotics for infections, possible surgical drainage of abscess, and surgical correction for anatomic problems such as strictures. Treat pain, as many of these inflammatory disorders are extremely painful. If sepsis occurs, must be hospitalized. Use warm or cold compresses and scrotal support if indicated.

Nursing Interventions and Complications

Patient education focusing on measures to reduce discomfort from swelling and pain, and alleviate systemic symptoms. Warm or cold compresses or a scrotal support may be used. Bed rest may be indicated for these conditions in the acute phase, sitz baths, give analgesics/antipyretics and stool softeners to avoid straining during bowel movement causing further pain, give antibiotics as ordered. Give emotional support and allow the man to verbalize his fears surrounding fertility and/or chronic pain and spasms.

CLINICAL ALERT

Urinary strictures as a result of the inflammatory process can impede urination and lead to kidney failure. Orchitis can lead to fibrosis of the testicle and if both testicles are involved the patient would be infertile. Nurses should educate young men about the results of STIs and the pain men suffer.

CASE STUDY

SL is a 29-year-old woman with very irregular periods and often does not get a period for 6–7 months, and to get a period she must be induced to get a bleed because of the high risk of endometrial cancer. She is obese and has hair on her chin (which she shaves) and on her chest and also has facial acne. She has met a man and would like to get pregnant and worries about this. She is put on metformin, loses some weight, and begins somewhat regular menses. On sonogram, it does not indicate that SL is ovulating. The man she met, MS, had inflammation and infection in both his testicles when he was 17 years old due to a virus and he believes he is infertile.

QUESTIONS

1. What syndrome is SL suffering with?
2. What hormones are elevated to cause her symptoms?
3. What medication can she be given to try to stimulate ovulation?
4. What virus did MS suffer with that would leave him infertile?
5. (a) What test would be ordered to determine if SL is ovulating and what (b) test would determine if MS was infertile?

Suggested Readings

Bensen S, Hahn S, Tan S, Janssen OF, Schedlowski M, Elsenbruch S. Maladaptive coping with illness in women with polycystic ovary syndrome. *J Obstet Gynecol Neonatal Nurs.* 2010;39(1):37-45.

Brill JR. Diagnosis and treatment of urethritis in men. *Am Fam Physician.* 2010; 8(7):873-878.

Burton ME, Daley AM. Health-risk counseling for adolescents with polycystic ovary syndrome. *Am J Nurse Pract.* 2011;15:51-60.

Domino FW, ed. *The 5-Minute Clinical Consult 2011.* 19th ed. Philadelphia, PA: Wolters Kluwer/Lippincott Williams & Wilkins; 2010.

Fantansia HC, Fontenot HB, Sutherland M, Harris AL. Sexually transmitted infections in women. *Nurs Womens Health.* 2011;15(1):46-57.

Fontenot HB, Morelock N. HPV in men is a women's health issue. *Nurs Womens Health.* 2012;16(1):57-65.

Kieliszek K. Trends in microbial resistance: treating *Neisseria gonorrhoeae* infection. *Am J Nurse Pract.* 2011;15(9/10):8-12.

Montplaisir P. Is metformin a multifunctional medication for inducing ovulation and improving pregnancy outcomes in PCOS? *J Am Acad Nurse Pract.* 2011;11(16): 537-541.

Peters RM. High blood pressure in pregnancy. *Nurs Womens Health.* 2008;12(5):410-421.

Phipps WJ, Monhahan FD, Sands JK, Marek JF, Neighbors M. *Medical-Surgical Nursing Health and Illness Perspectives.* 7th ed. St. Louis, MO: Mosby; 2003.

Ricci SS, Kyle T. *Maternity and Pediatric Nursing.* Philadelphia, PA: Wolters Kluwer/ Lippincott Williams & Wilkins; 2009.

Roe AH, Dokras A. The diagnosis of polycystic ovary syndrome. *Obstet Gynecol.* 2011;4(2):45-51.

Story L. *Pathophysiology: A Practical Approach.* Sudbury, MA: Jones & Bartlett; 2012.

Taber's Cyclopedic Medical Dictionary. Philadelphia, PA: F.A. Davis; 2009.

Townsend MC. *Psychiatric Mental Health Nursing.* 5th ed. Philadelphia, PA: F.A. Davis; 2006.

Watkins J. Mumps: an overview of the diagnosis and complications. *Br J Sch Nurs.* 2011;6(2):73-76.

Weiss TR, Bilmer SM. Young women's experiences living with polycystic ovary syndrome. *J Obstet Gynecol Neonatal Nurs.* 2011;40(6):709-718.

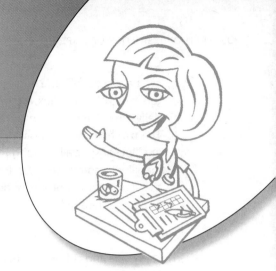

Answers

CASE STUDY ANSWERS

CHAPTER 1

1. Memory loss, feelings of anxiety and paranoia, elevated blood pressure, inappropriate orientation, thoughts of misplacing or theft of personal effects, forgetfulness
2. Fall risk, medication safety, cognitive decline
3. The planned discharge is safe for this patient. The continuous aide in the home monitoring of the patient as well as weekly visits from the nurse assure medication compliance, safety, and monitoring of the patient. The ultimate goal is to keep the patient out of the hospital.
4. Vital signs, nutrition, physical mobility, safety with medications, complication prevention, and timely healthcare provider visits.
5. Keeping medications in a safe place. Keeping walking area clear of clutter. Proper nutrition and hydration to prevent weight loss, muscle mass loss, weakened bones, and dehydration

CHAPTER 2

1. Target system: Respiratory. The presentation of pneumonia (PNA) common among the geriatric patients warrants prompt assessment and interventions to prevent complications such as respiratory failure/arrest and or septicemia.
2. Airway management takes priority with this patient followed by hydration via IV fluids.
3. Antibiotic treatment via IV infusion tapering to PO as patient progresses. IV hydration, antipyretics for fever if necessary, small frequent meals for added nutrition, HOB 45°, possible oxygen via nasal cannula, nebulizer treatments, and incentive spirometry.
4. Three priority outcomes: resolution of pneumonia, prevention of decompensation: nutrition/hydration, home discharge
5. Two possible complications: progression of disease process leading to respiratory failure and generalized weakness that can lead to aspiration. Avoidance of these two complications

can be successful if the nurse maintains hand hygiene, monitors vital signs as ordered, monitors patient's gag reflex, listens to lung and heart sounds, has the patient sit up when eating, delivering all medication correctly and timely and monitoring for complications.

6. The psychological complications could be anxiety and/or depression. Chronic or debilitating illness especially among the elderly can potentiate feelings of loss if independence and inability to complete ADLs. Patients can become depressed quickly. Nurses need to know the signs and symptoms of depression and assist the patient and their family by referring patients as needed.

CHAPTER 3

1. Language and cultural norms are two major barriers.
2. The nurse should set time up on the next appointment to review all the medications and take the time to educate the patient on medications and importance of follow-through with medications and follow-up appointments.
3. Make weekly appointments times 4 weeks to monitor blood pressure.
4. It is difficult to say if the blood pressure medication is not working as the patient is known to have poor compliance with medications. Weekly monitoring should provide a better sense of medication appropriateness and its response on blood pressure measurements.
5. Take the medication as ordered, do not stop taking the medication as your blood pressure stabilizes, and follow up on weekly appointments.
6. Weekly
7. Blood work, urinalysis & proteinuria, renal scan (r/o renal artery stenosis), CRP, homocysteine level, CPK

CHAPTER 4

1. Ulcerative colitis
2. Stop smoking and refer to smoking cessation clinic
3. Gall stones or sludge (cholecystitis)
4. Ultrasonography, CT, Endoscopic surgery
5. Peptic ulcer, gastritis, hepatitis, pancreatitis, gallbladder cancer

CHAPTER 5

1. Elevated fasting blood sugars, elevated HgA1C, frequent thirst, urination and hunger, high carb diet, and fatigue
2. Burning, pins and needles feeling in the feet, and cold intolerance
3. Glucosuria, parethesia in extremities, diminishing vision
4. Weight loss, increasing exercise and diet/nutrition
5. Obesity as her BMI is >30 and possible metabolic syndrome

CHAPTER 6

1. Interstitial cystitis
2. Symptoms that food and diet can make worse, and irritation inside the bladder on direct visualization doing a cystoscopy.

3. Nursing diagnosis is pain and the nurse would assess what the patient's diet is to determine if symptoms increase with certain foods.
4. A negative urine culture and sensitivity and cytology
5. Elmiron PO (orally), TID (twice daily)

CHAPTER 7

1. Additional work-up includes recommendations from the American College of Rheumatology: joint involvements, serology: RF, ACPA, ESR and CRP, and symptom duration
2. Rheumatology
3. NSAIDS may be started at low dose for symptom management but patient should be referred to rheumatology as soon as possible.
4. If possible, patients can be started on DMARDS as soon as rheumatoid arthritis criteria have been met.
5. As with all NSAIDS, gastric upset and ulcer formation and bleeding are important complications to monitor patients. DMARDS lower the immune response; therefore, patients are at a higher risk for the development of certain types of cancers and infections.
6. Development of nodules, joint movement limitation or freezing, gait disturbance, loss of motor skills, and falls

CHAPTER 8

1. Primary diagnosis: poison ivy
2. Secondary diagnosis: contact dermatitis, cellulitis
3. Wash site with cold water and soap as soon as possible. Washing immediately after significantly reduces the incidence of further progression. Use cold water because warm water allows urishiol, the ingredient of the plant that causes skin problems, to penetrate into the skin quicker. Topical steroids of lowest potency for mild dermatitis, moving to higher potency for more severe dermatitis. With severe dermatitis, oral steroids might be necessary. Antihistamines are useful to relieve the itching.
4. Follow-up within 7-10 days after treatments has started.
5. Wear long sleeves and long pants when in the yard to prevent exposure. Use of barrier over-the-counter creams; get prompt treatment to avoid complications such as cellulitis

CHAPTER 11

1. She has never been pregnant (nulliparity), eats a diet high in fat, is sedentary, and has many years of uninterrupted hormones due to early age of period and is still menstruating (37 years).
2. Is there a family history of breast cancer and if so, what ages were the relatives with breast cancer? What is her normal menstrual cycle?
3. The upper outer quadrant of the breast.
4. First the nurse practitioner would examine the lump and arrange for a mammography, breast sonogram, and a stereotactic biopsy or fine-needle biopsy.
5. Because the patient's husband found the lump, the nurse practitioner should reinforce self breast examination, decrease fats in the diet and eat fruits and vegetables, begin an exercise program and concentrate on losing weight. The patient must have at least annual complete physicals, including blood work and an annual Pap test and a mammogram.

CHAPTER 13

1. PCOS (Polycystic ovarian syndrome)
2. Androgens or testosterone
3. Clomid
4. Mumps
5. (a) Sonogram to determine if dominant follicle or hormone testing
   (b) Sperm analysis

REVIEW ANSWERS

CHAPTER 7

1. **B**
2. **D**
3. **A**

CHAPTER 9

1. **A**
2. **D**

CHAPTER 10

1. **C.** Listening to lung sounds is priority as the registered nurse determines the respiratory status of the patient and the presence or absence of any adventitious breath sounds that can impair oxygenation.
2. **A.** A patient in sickle cell crisis requires immediate pain management. IV medications are chosen for their quick onset of action. Although the other measures are also part of the patient assessment and interventions process, starting the IV access for medication administration for effective pain relief is priority.
3. **A.** A patient who has a compromised immune systems such as the one with leukemia requires protection. Reverse isolation prevents the introduction of infections by health care personnel and visitors effectively. While the patient may suffer from social isolation, the priority remains protection from infection.
4. **C.** The Z-track method prevents or reduces leakage of medication through subcutaneous tissue, thus avoiding a reduced dose and reducing the incidence of skin trauma.
5. **D.** The immune-compromised patient must be protected. Frequent and consistent hand washing, eating well-cooked foods, and eliminating live plants will help keep the patient safe from breaks in the chain of infection.

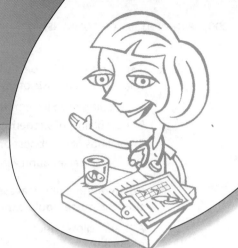

Final Exam Questions

1. A client has been admitted to the burn unit with extensive full-thickness burns. Which of the following considerations has priority?

   A. Fluid status
   B. Body image
   C. Level of pain
   D. Risk of infection

2. A client is admitted to the hospital with respiratory difficulty, wheezing on expiration, coughing, and diaphoresis. An intravenous infusion of aminophylline is ordered. The nurse knows that one of the following best describes the purpose of giving this medication:

   A. To relax the bronchial smooth muscles
   B. To increase the tone in the respiratory passages
   C. To cause bronchoconstriction
   D. To decrease the inflammatory reaction

3. A 74-year-old client is admitted with respiratory acidosis as a complication of chronic obstructive pulmonary disorder (COPD). Her blood gases reveal she is in primary respiratory acidosis. The nurse knows that this probably results from:

   A. Increased mucous secretions
   B. Decreased exhalation of carbon dioxide
   C. Long-term theophylline administration
   D. Recent vomiting and diarrhea

4. The nurse would expect to make which of the following observations about a client to relate to a diagnosis of myocardial infarction rather than angina?

   A. A feeling of an intermittent strangling sensation

   B. Complaints of sudden substernal pain after an argument

   C. Feelings of numbness or weakness in the arms or wrists

   D. Profuse perspiration with nausea and vomiting

5. When doing a physical assessment on a client with early common bile duct obstruction, the nurse would expect to see which clinical manifestation?

   A. Dark yellow urine

   B. Ascites

   C. Clay-colored feces

   D. Petechiae

6. A client is admitted to the hospital after complaining of chest pain. The client's history reveals congestive heart failure. He has been receiving digoxin (Lanoxin). The nurse understands that the purpose of giving the client digoxin is to:

   A. Increase cardiac size

   B. Decrease cardiac output

   C. Increase the force of cardiac contraction

   D. Slow the pulse rate

7. A common nursing diagnosis for a client in the immediate postoperative phase after a TURP (transurethral resection of the prostate gland) is:

   A. Ineffective peripheral tissue perfusions related to deep vein thrombosis

   B. Altered comfort related to pain of bladder spasms

   C. Disturbed body image related to disfiguring surgery

   D. Imbalanced nutrition: less than body requirements

8. A client asks the nurse, "Where is cancer usually found in the breast?" When responding to the client, the nurse uses a diagram of a left breast and indicates that the most malignant tumors occur in the:

   A. Upper outer quadrant

   B. Upper inner quadrant

   C. Lower outer quadrant

   D. Lower inner quadrant

9. The primary function of the prostate gland is:

   A. To store underdeveloped sperm before ejaculation

   B. To regulate the acidity and alkalinity of the environment for proper sperm development

   C. To produce a secretion that aids the nourishment and passage of sperm

   D. To secrete a hormone that stimulates the production and maturation of sperm

10. **The client with hypertension is prone to long-term complications of the disease. Which of the following is a long-term complication of hypertension?**

    A. Renal insufficiency and failure

    B. Valvular heart disease

    C. Endocarditis

    D. Peptic ulcer disease

11. **The nurse is caring for a client who is undergoing chemotherapy. Current laboratory values include:**

    A. Hemoglobin 12.0 mg/dl

    B. Hematocrit 34%

    C. Platelet count 108,000/mm³

    D. White blood cell (WBC) 1,600/mm³ and absolute neutrophil count is calculated to be <1.000/mm³

12. **Which of the sign(s) and/or symptoms would be observed in a client with hypoglycemia and impending insulin shock? Check all that apply.**

    A. Rapid, shallow respirations

    B. Fetid breath odor

    C. Irritability

    D. Confusion

    E. Clammy skin

    F. Slurring of words

13. **The client with Addison disease is taking glucocorticoids at home. Which of the following statements correctly reflects the principle governing administration and dosage of glucocorticoids?**

    A. Various circumstances increase the need for glucocorticoids, so dosage adjustments will be needed.

    B. The need for glucocorticoids stabilizes, and a predetermined dose is taken once a day.

    C. Glucocorticoids are cumulative, so a dose is taken every third day.

    D. A dose is taken every 6 hours to ensure consistent blood levels of glucocorticoids.

14. **The nurse evaluates the client's most recent laboratory data. Which laboratory findings would be consistent with a diagnosis of acute pancreatitis?**

    A. Hyperglycemia

    B. Leukopenia

    C. Thrombocytopenia

    D. Hyperkalemia

15. Atherosclerosis results in stenosis of the arteries. Which of the following vascular problems is also a result of atherosclerosis?

A. Thickened endothelial lining of the vessel walls

B. Formation of an aneurysm

C. Hardening of the arteries

D. Formation of varicose veins

16. The nurse is admitting a 69-year-old to the clinical unit. The client has a history of left ventricular enlargement. During assessment, the nurse notes 3+ pitting edema of the ankles bilaterally. The client does not have chest pain. The nurse observes that the client does have dyspnea at rest. The nurse infers that the client may have:

A. Arteriosclerosis

B. Heart failure

C. Chronic bronchitis

D. Acute myocardial infarction

17. A 28-year-old male client is diagnosed with acute epididymitis. The nurse would expect to find that the symptoms that caused the client to seek medical care are:

A. Burning and pain on urination

B. Severe tenderness and swelling of the scrotum

C. Foul-smelling ejaculate

D. Foul-smelling urine

18. When educating a female client with gonorrhea, the nurse should emphasize that for women gonorrhea:

A. Is often marked by symptoms of dysuria or vaginal bleeding

B. Does not lead to serious complications

C. Can be treated but not cured

D. May not cause symptoms until serious complications occur

19. The nurse evaluates the client correctly understands how to report signs of bleeding when she makes which of the following statements:

A. "Petechiae are large red skin bruises"

B. "Ecchymoses are large purple skin bruises"

C. "Purpura is an open cut on the skin"

D. "Abrasions are small pinpoint red dots on the skin"

20. A client with gastroesophageal reflux disease (GERD) complains of a chronic cough. The nurse understands that a client with this symptom of GERD may indicate which of the following?

A. Development of laryngeal cancer

B. Irritation of the esophagus

   C. Esophageal scar tissue formation

   D. Aspiration of gastric contents

21. **Which of the following clients are at greatest risk for developing acute renal failure?**

   A. A dialysis client who gets influenza

   B. A teenager who has an appendectomy

   C. A pregnant woman who has a fractured femur

   D. A client with diabetes who has a heart catheterization

22. **During the initial stage of burns, a primary fluid imbalance occurs. The nurse knows there has been a shift of fluids from:**

   A. The cell to interstitial space

   B. The interstitial space to the cell

   C. The interstitial space to the plasma

   D. The plasma to the interstitial space

23. **The nurse would be correct in saying the two most common causes of hypothyroidism are:**

   A. Destruction of thyroid tissue by radioactive iodine during therapy for hyperthyroidism and spontaneous atrophy due to autoimmune response

   B. Spontaneous atrophy due to autoimmune response and surgical removal of the thyroid gland

   C. Surgical removal of the thyroid gland, and tumors of the pituitary gland that decrease the circulating amount of thyroxine

   D. Tumors of the pituitary gland and/or large doses of antithyroid drugs

24. **Because aldosterone is the major mineralocorticoid secreted by the adrenal cortex, which fluid and electrolyte imbalance should the nurse anticipate with decreased secretion of this hormone?**

   A. Hyperkalemia

   B. Hypernatremia

   C. Hypervolemia

   D. Hypercalcemia

25. **A client returns from surgery for her fractured hip. Her family is waiting anxiously to see her. What is the most important parameter for the nurse to assess immediately after the client is transferred to her bed?**

   A. The client's ability to deep breathe and cough

   B. The client's vital signs

   C. The surgical dressing

   D. Turn the client on the unaffected side

26. Following a spinal cord injury at or above T6, the nurse should watch the client closely for signs of autonomic dysreflexia. The nurse is aware that this potentially dangerous response could be triggered by:

   A. Elevated blood pressure

   B. Severe headache

   C. Distended bladder

   D. Edema of the spinal cord

27. A 92-year-old client is admitted to the hospital with abdominal pain. During the initial assessment, the nurse notes that the client is not giving appropriate answers to questions. The client just nods and smiles while the nurse is talking to him. The nurse is probably dealing with what developmental problem?

   A. The client is experiencing so much pain that he cannot focus on the nurse's questions.

   B. It must be assumed that the client is probably confused at his age

   C. The client is probably hard of hearing

   D. Most elderly live in a fantasy world and are unable to comprehend what others say to them

28. Four days after admission for cirrhosis of the liver, a client began to bleed from an esophageal varix. The earliest indications of bleeding noted by the nurse would include:

   A. Tachycardia, restlessness, and pallor

   B. Tachycardia, lethargy, and flushing

   C. Sudden drop in blood pressure of 10 mm Hg or more

   D. Increasing combativeness and widening pulse pressure

29. Admitted to the hospital with pulmonary emphysema, a client is extremely short of breath and is receiving oxygen per nasal cannula. The most important nursing action for this client receiving oxygen therapy is to:

   A. Make sure the client is receiving at least 6 L

   B. Provide low oxygen percentages to prevent respiratory arrest

   C. Provide oral hygiene

   D. Clean nostrils around the cannula as needed

30. A client is admitted to the hospital with respiratory difficulty, wheezing on expiration, coughing, and diaphoresis. An intravenous infusion of aminophylline is ordered. The nurse knows that one of the following best describes the purpose of ordering this medication:

   A. To relax the bronchial smooth muscle

   B. To increase the tone in the respiratory passages

   C. To cause bronchoconstriction

   D. To decrease the inflammatory reaction

31. A client diagnosed with urolithiasis is advised to follow a low-calcium diet after pathology report reveals calcium oxalate stones. Which of the following four selections indicates to the nurse the need for further teaching?

    A. Hamburger, baked potato, squash
    B. Shrimp, scalloped potatoes, broccoli
    C. Chicken, wild rice, green beans
    D. Roast pork, whipped potatoes, carrots

32. A client who has been diagnosed with congestive heart failure (CHF) two days earlier begins to exhibit symptoms of left-sided heart failure. Which of the following would the nurse observe?

    A. Peripheral edema
    B. Dyspnea
    C. Abdominal distention
    D. Fatigue

33. The nurse assists an asthmatic client with a face mask delivering humidified oxygen at 35%. The nurse knows that the effectiveness of this therapy is best demonstrated by:

    A. Absence of adventitious breath sounds
    B. Pao_2 of 92
    C. Heart rate increase of 25 beats/min
    D. Bicarbonate level of 25 mEq/L

34. A client is admitted with acute leukemia. The nurse can anticipate that the client will report which of the following clusters of symptoms?

    A. Nausea/vomiting, diarrhea
    B. Fatigue, weakness
    C. Fever, chills
    D. Nosebleed, headache

35. A client, age 26, has been diagnosed with AIDS and is currently hospitalized for treatment of *Pneumocystis carinii* pneumonia. Which of the following symptoms would the nurse expect to observe with a client with this type of pneumonia?

    A. Hemoptysis
    B. Fever
    C. General malaise
    D. Dyspnea

36. The most important nursing goal for a client who is admitted with acute exacerbation of ulcerative colitis is at which of the following?

    A. To provide emotional support
    B. To prevent skin breakdown

C. To maintain fluid and electrolyte balance

D. To promote physical rest

37. **Second- and third-degree burns of the head, neck, and chest place the client initially at greatest risk for which of the following?**

A. Infection

B. Airway obstruction

C. Fluid imbalance

D. Paralytic ileus

38. **The nurse would expect the client with hyperthyroidism to report which of the following?**

A. Weight gain of 10 lbs in 3 weeks

B. Constipation

C. Sensitivity to cold

D. Flushed, moist skin

39. **When assessing a client with glaucoma, a nurse expects which of the following?**

A. Complaints of double vision

B. Complaints of halos around the lights

C. Intraocular pressure of 15 mm Hg

D. Soft globe on palpation

40. **Which of the following conditions or actions can cause primary osteoarthritis?**

A. Overuse of joints, aging, obesity

B. Obesity, diabetes mellitus, aging

C. Congenital abnormality, aging, overuse of joints

D. Diabetes mellitus, congenital abnormality, aging

41. **A 19-year-old client is admitted with heat stroke and begins to show signs of disseminated intravascular coagulation (DIC). Which of the following laboratory findings is most consistent with DIC?**

A. Low platelet count

B. Elevated fibrinogen levels

C. Low levels of fibrin degradation products

D. Reduced prothrombin time

42. **Copious amounts of frothy, greenish vaginal discharge would be a symptom of which of the following?**

A. Candidiasis

B. *Gardnerella vaginalis* vaginitis

C. Gonorrhea

D. Trichomoniasis

43. Which of the following characteristics is typical of the pain associated with deep vein thrombosis (DVT)?

    A. Dull ache

    B. No pain

    C. Sudden onset

    D. Tingling

44. Which of the following assessment findings indicates an increased risk for skin cancer?

    A. A deep sunburn

    B. A dark mole on the patient's back

    C. An irregular scar on the client's abdomen

    D. White irregular patches on the client's arm

45. Scoliosis can be described by which of the following definitions?

    A. An increase in the lumbar curve

    B. A decrease in the thoracic kyphosis

    C. Lateral curves in the spinal column described as right or left concavities

    D. Lateral curves in the spinal column described as right or left convexities

46. Sickle-cell anemia occurs primarily in which of the following ethnic groups?

    A. African American

    B. Asian

    C. Hispanic

    D. Caucasian

47. A nurse is caring for a client who recently underwent surgery for a fractured radius and ulna after a motor vehicle accident. Which action should the nurse include in a care plan for a client with a fiberglass case on the right arm?

    A. Keep the casted arm warm with a light blanket

    B. Avoid handling the cast for 24 hours or until dry

    C. Assess dorsalis pedis and posterior tibial pulses every 2 hours

    D. Assess movement and sensation in the fingers of the right hand

48. A client with Addison disease has been admitted to the nursing unit with dehydration. Your initial assessment confirms a nursing diagnosis of deficient fluid volume. Which etiologic factor establishes this nursing diagnosis?

    A. Glucocorticoid excess

    B. Mineralocorticoid deficiency

    C. Melanocyte-stimulating hormone excess

    D. Melanocyte-stimulating hormone deficit

49. A nurse is reviewing the laboratory results of a client with rheumatoid arthritis. Which laboratory result should the nurse expect to find?

A. Increased platelet count

B. Elevated erythrocyte sedimentation rate (ERS)

C. Electrolyte imbalance

D. Altered blood urea nitrogen (BUN) and creatinine levels

50. A nurse is caring for a client with a fractured hip. The client is combative and confused and he's trying to get out of bed. The nurse should:

A. Leave the client and get help

B. Obtain a physician's order to restrain the client

C. Read the facility's policy on restraints

D. Order soft restraints from the storeroom

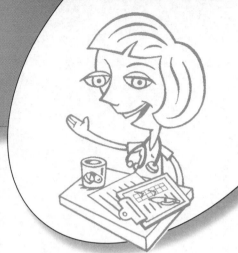

Final Exam Answers

1. A
2. A
3. B
4. D
5. C
6. C
7. B
8. A
9. C
10. A
11. D
12. A, C, E, F
13. A
14. A
15. B
16. B
17. B
18. D
19. B
20. D
21. D
22. A
23. A
24. A
25. B

26. C
27. C
28. A
29. B
30. A
31. B
32. B
33. B
34. B
35. A
36. C
37. B
38. D
39. B
40. A
41. A
42. D
43. C
44. A
45. D
46. A
47. D
48. B
49. B
50. B

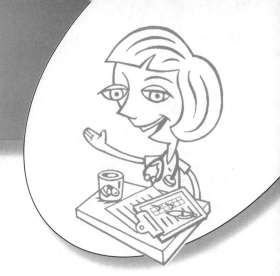

Index

Note: Page numbers followed by *f* denote figures; page numbers followed by *t* denote tables.